The Sinus Sourcebook

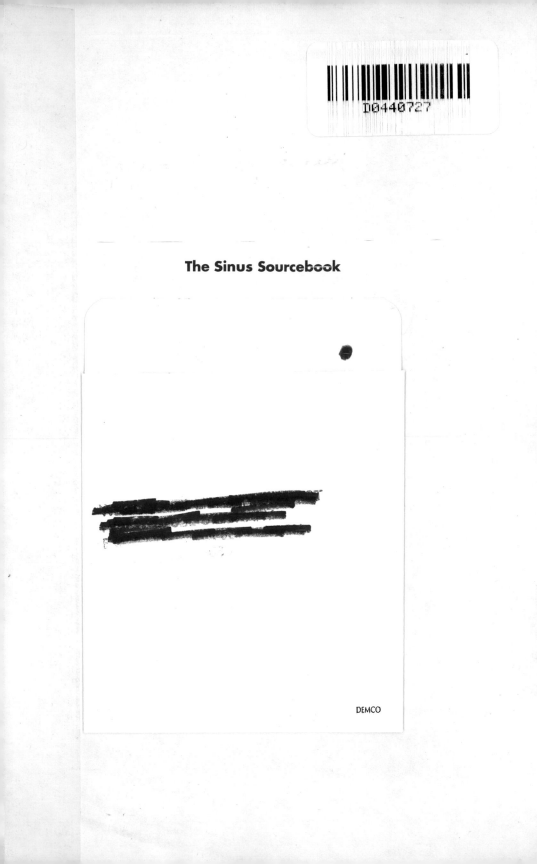

THE SINUS
SOURCEBOOK

by

Deborah Rosin, M.D.

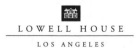

LOWELL HOUSE

LOS ANGELES

CONTEMPORARY BOOKS

CHICAGO

NOTICE: The author and publisher of this book have, as far as it is possible to do so, taken care to make certain that recommendations regarding the treatment and use of drugs are correct and compatible with the
standards generally accepted at the time of publication. However,
knowledge in medical science is constantly changing. As new information becomes available, changes in treatment and in the use of drugs
may become necessary. The reader is urged to consult his or her physician for professional advice in dealing with any serious or potentially
serious medical problem.

Library of Congress Cataloging-in-Publication Data

Rosin, Deborah.
    The sinus sourcebook / by Deborah Rosin.
        p. cm.
    Includes bibliographical references and index.
    ISBN 1-56565-643-1
    ISBN 0-7373-0083-3 (paper edition)
    1. Paranasal sinuses—Diseases.   2. Sinusitis.   I. Title.
    RF421.r67   1998
    617.5'23—dc21
                                                              97-50154
                                                              CIP

Requests for such permissions should be addressed to:
Lowell House
2020 Avenue of the Stars, Suite 300
Los Angeles, CA 90067

Lowell House books can be purchased at special discounts when
ordered in bulk for premiums and special sales.

Publisher: Jack Artenstein
Associate Publisher, Lowell House Adult: Bud Sperry
Director of Publishing Services: Rena Copperman
Managing Editor: Maria Magallanes
Text design: Laurie Young
Illustrations courtesy of Deborah Rosin and Elizabeth Weadon Massari

Printed and bound in the United States of America
10 9 8 7 6 5 4 3 2

To my father

CONTENTS

FOREWORD

This self-help book was written in response to several major trends in medicine. Any experienced physician knows that prevention of an illness is the best cure. By understanding the factors that contribute to your sinus problems, you can hopefully avoid or at least minimize them. Among the most common illnesses for which people seek medical advice are colds, allergies, and sinus ailments. All of these subjects are explained in easily understood terms in the chapters that follow. Many of the symptoms associated with these illnesses can be relieved with self-help measures. With the increasing number of medications now available without a prescription, consumers need an understanding of which products are effective and which should be avoided. Unfortunately, many widely advertised "sinus products" may be inappropriate. The chapter on medications explains how to select nonprescription medications for optimal relief of your symptoms. While many nasal and sinus problems lend themselves to simple solutions, some progress or recur to the point that make evaluation and treatment by a physician necessary. An understanding of factors that may be contributing to these illnesses will enable you to present pertinent background information to your physician, improving the chance of an effective treatment program. Since many of the illnesses covered in this book also affect children, parents will find many suggestions to help recognize problems and provide relief until medical help can be obtained. For the vast number of people affected by disorders of the nose and sinuses, this book should provide a lot of helpful and practical information to start them on the road to recovery.

—STANLEY N. FARB, M.D.

INTRODUCTION TO THE SINUSES

A s an ear, nose, and throat doctor, I see at least five patients a day who tell me that they have "sinus trouble." Take, for example, Jesse, a twenty-five-year-old woman who had suffered through one week of pressure in her cheeks and forehead, thick, yellow mucus coming from her nose, and clogging of her ears. Despite using over-the-counter drugs, she still couldn't breathe out of her nose and had touble making it through a day of work. After ten days of using a prescription antibiotic and an oral decongestant, she was back to normal and never had another nasal problem for years.

Joe, on the other hand, was a forty-year-old marketing executive who, after moving to an old farmhouse near Princeton, New Jersey, began noticing "sinus problems" of facial pressure and headache. In addition, he had resumed smoking because of the increased pressures at work. When allergy-testing revealed that he was a highly allergic individual, he made his home as dust free as possible and put in an air-filtering system. When he was also able to quit smoking, his headaches subsided.

Jeff, an otherwise healthy five year old, was brought in by his parents because of his "sinuses." He had a constant runny nose and deep cough despite many months of different medications from his pediatrician. Once his adenoids were removed and his sinuses drained, his breathing and nasal problems normalized.

These are just three examples of the many ways that sinus problems can present and be treated. Jesse had an acute, short-lived sinus infection that responded well to medical treatment. Joe's sinus problems had a strong allergy component that needed to be adressed for ultimate resolution of his symptoms. And Jeff 's was a case of childhood sinusitis. These three, like another 30 to 35 million Americans, have "sinus problems." In fact, sinus symptoms are one of the most common complaints that leads a patient to a doctor's office. Roughly 20 million office visits occur in the United States yearly because of sinus disease, resulting in 16 million prescriptions written each year.

Before we can discuss sinus disorders and their treatment, we must first understand what sinuses are and how they function. What happens in the sinus is often closely related to the nose, so nasal function will also be considered.

THE SINUSES—
WHAT THEY ARE AND WHAT THEY DO

Most people who complain about their sinuses are talking about their "paranasal sinuses." These are air-filled bony cavities that are located adjacent to the nose in the face and skull. They are lined by membranes that are similar to those which line the nose. Each sinus is connected into the nose by a small opening called an ostium. The sinuses begin in babies as small pockets the size of a pea and grow through childhood to adult size—about the size of a walnut.

There are four sets of paired sinuses, as shown in Figures 1.1 and 1.2.

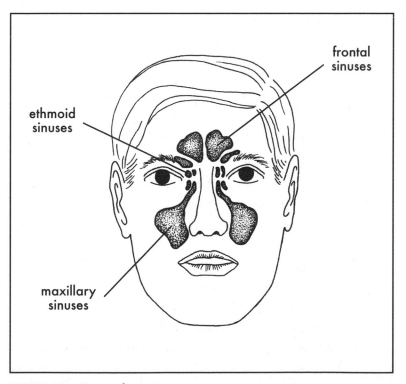

FIGURE 1.1   Sinuses, front view.

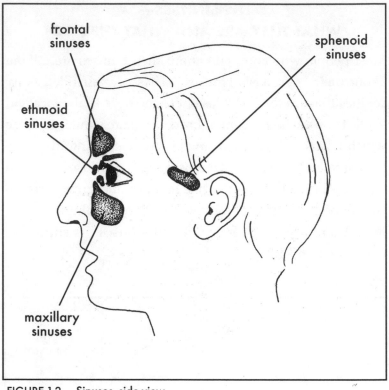

FIGURE 1.2   Sinuses, side view.

1. **frontal sinuses**—sit in the forehead
2. **maxillary sinuses**—sit in the cheek above the teeth and below the eyes
3. **ethmoid sinuses**—sit on each side of the nose between the eyes
4. **sphenoid sinuses**—sit behind the eyes, and are the most deeply placed

Sometimes the sinuses can differ in size from one side to the other. Some people may be missing one sinus in the pair, but this rarely causes a problem. This asymmetry is most often seen with the frontal sinus.

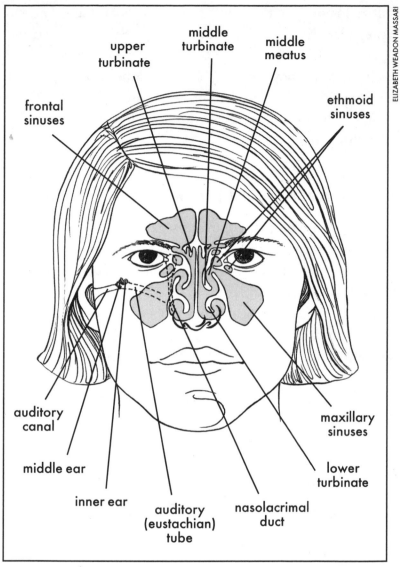

FIGURE 1.3   The sinuses.

Despite all we know about the sinuses, there is still some debate regarding their purpose. Some people believe that they lighten your dense skull. Another theory is that they aid in voice resonance, which is one reason physicians often do not want to operate on professional singers' noses: They fear changing their vocal quality. Some feel that the sinuses regulate pressure inside the nose, while others believe that they act as shock absorbers during head trauma. (A medical student once told me that the primary purpose of the sinuses is to provide a living for ear, nose, and throat doctors.)

THE NOSE—WHAT IT IS AND WHAT IT DOES

On page 5 is a diagram of the nose (Figure 1.3).

The partition that separates the right and left sides of the nose is called the *septum*. It is made up of cartilage in the front and of bone farther back. Often, a person has a deviated septum, which means they have a twist of the septum. If this deviation occurs to a significant degree, it may result in nasal blockage and even affect sinus drainage.

There are bones on the sidewall of the nose called *turbinates*. There are three turbinates on each side of the nose. The tear duct from the eye (called the nasolacrimal duct) drains underneath the lower, or inferior turbinate. This is why women may see coloring from their eye-lining pencil in their nasal drainage. The middle turbinate is the most important, since it is where the maxillary and anterior ethmoid sinuses drain. The posterior ethmoid and the sphenoid sinus drain under the upper, or superior turbinate, into the nose.

The back of the nose is called the *nasopharynx*. The *eustachian tube* runs between the nasopharynx and the ear, equalizing pressures between them. When a person has nasal or sinus problems, this leads to inflammation of the nasopharynx in the back of the nose, eventually causing a feeling of clogged ears. Additionally, tumors of the nasopharynx, which block the eustachian tube opening, prevent adequate ear drainage and ventilation, resulting in fluid behind the eardrum.

The tissue that sits in the nasopharynx is called *adenoid* tissue. It is made up of lymph tissue, which helps fight infection (this function of adenoid tissue is only important clinically during the first year of life). Adenoid tissue is present in children and tends to shrink during the late teen years and early twenties. Large adenoids can lead to blockage of sinus drainage and sinus disease. In the past, large adenoids were treated by radium, but this has led to increased cancer rates, and so today, large adenoids are surgically removed.

Your nose does a lot more than just fill up the middle of your face. Its primary functions are respiration and smell. While respiration, or breathing, can be carried out via the mouth, it is the nose that is uniquely suited to this function. As air is drawn into the nose for ultimate passage to the lungs, it must be cleaned of the microscopic particles we inhale. These include dust, pollen, and the many pollutants of an industrialized society. The small hairs inside the nose, called cilia, as well as nasal mucus carry out this cleaning process. The nose not only acts as nature's vacuum cleaner, but it is also a humidifier and temperature regulator. Think about when you go outside on a very cold day. If that sub-zero air got through to your lungs, it would cause serious damage. Your nose and respiratory system warm the air to body temperature, protecting the sensitive lining of the lungs and bronchial tubes.

Most people breathe through their nose when they can. When your nose is blocked (see Chapter 4), you have to switch to breathing through your mouth. This can cause problems:

- When you breathe primarily through your mouth, for instance, when you have a cold, you may end up with a sore throat. This is because the nose humidifies the air you breathe, keeping your throat from getting too dry.

- Sometimes people snore because they are unable to breathe through their nose.

- When mouth breathing persists for a long time (several years), it may lead to a dull facial expression. This is called "adenoid facies" in children when it is due to large adenoids.

- Newborns breathe exclusively through their noses. This becomes important during eating, when the mouth is full. Thus, anything that blocks the nose in a newborn will lead to the inability to breathe during eating, and so must be attended to promptly.

Your nose also keeps diseases out of your body. Since viruses and bacteria often enter the body through the upper respiratory tract (nose and throat), the nasal lining and mucus that coat the tract act as our first line of defense. In some people, the process of filtering out dust and disease triggers an "allergic reaction." Later, in Chapter 5, we will take an in-depth look at allergy as it relates to nose and sinus disease.

The other important function of the nose is smell. The medical term for smell is *olfaction.* While humans have a less developed sense of smell than some other animals, our ability to smell still accounts for important responses, such as appetite and emotion. Think about all the ways that your sense of smell affects your life:

- When you're an infant, you sense the nearness of your mother, in part, through smell, triggering the sucking response.

- When you smell food, it stimulates your appetite, ensuring that you eat and remain healthy.

- Conversely, foul-smelling items often signal rotten food, which protects you from eating them.

- Pleasant smells, such as perfume, or the absence of unpleasant smells, such as underarm odor, are the basis of multimillion-dollar businesses. Through the centuries, people have known that the sense of smell is a key to attracting the opposite sex.

- Your sense of smell protects you from the dangers of fire and natural gas.

- Your sense of taste is closely linked to your sense of smell. You've probably noticed that when you have a bad cold and your nose is blocked, the taste of food is greatly diminished. Many people who complain about a change in taste are actually experiencing changes in their sense of smell. As people get older, their sense of smell decreases, leading to a decrease in appetite, which can become a medical problem, with significant associated weight loss.

You probably go through most days of your life never thinking about your sense of smell, when, in fact, it is an integral part of many things you do.

MUCUS OF THE NOSE AND SINUSES

Mucus is produced by glands within the lining of the nasal passages and sinus cavities. This mucus "blanket" serves a major role in the nasal defense mechanism by trapping foreign particles and organisms. The mucus contains a number of proteins and enzymes that can render these invaders harmless. Tiny hair cells, called cilia, move the mucus layer toward the back of the nose and throat, where the material is ultimately swallowed, for final deactivation by the stomach acids. The nose produces roughly a quart of mucus a day. Excessive or thickened mucus may result in plugging of the sinus openings with secondary infections. It also accounts for the postnasal drip, the feeling of mucus dripping down the back of the nose into the throat, which is common among sinus patients. I have seen some patients in which increased amounts of swallowed mucus can lead to nausea and vomiting. I even had a patient with colitis (intestinal disease), which only acted up when he had sinus infections.

In the past two decades, doctors have begun to better understand mucus drainage by using telescopes in the nose to follow drainage patterns. The wave of normal mucus production and flow within the sinuses into the nose is called mucociliary flow or mucociliary clearance. This refers to the movement of the mucus blanket on the cilia.

Mucus is directed from the maxillary and frontal sinuses toward an important area called the ostiomeatal complex (nicknamed the OMC). This OMC is primarily composed of ethmoid cells. Problems in the ethmoid sinus and the OMC lead to problems in the other sinuses, such as the frontal and the maxillary. In the past, the emphasis was placed on these secondarily infected frontal and maxillary sinuses. Currently, it is felt that the ethmoid sinuses and the OMC are the key to healthy sinuses, and by correcting drainage patterns here we can improve chronic sinus problems. This will be more fully addressed in Chapter 10, when we discuss the newer techniques of functional sinus surgery which normalize the sinuses to their proper function.

KEEPING SINUSES HEALTHY

A number of factors keep the sinuses healthy:

1. Sinuses stay healthy when their ostia (openings) are unblocked, allowing them to drain into the nose. If something is in the way of the normal drainage pattern, mucus is blocked which can lead to a sinus infection. Examples of things that can get in the way of normal drainage are swelling resulting from a typical cold or allergy; growths, such as polyps; or anatomic abnormalities, such as a deviated septum.

2. The mucus blanket must have normal contents and be of a normal amount. Part of what makes up the mucus blanket are enzymes that fight infection, and if these are missing, sinus infection may result. If there is an increase in mucus produced, this too can lead to infection.

3. Hair cells move mucus toward the sinus ostia. The interior of the nose is also lined by hair cells, which must be functioning normally to have proper sinus drainage. Anything that impairs the normal motion of hair cells may result in a nasal or sinus infection. For example, hair-cell motility is impaired in cystic

fibrosis sufferers. These patients are plagued with chronic sinus infections, as they are unable to normally clear the mucus in their nose and sinuses.

These three factors are interrelated. A problem in one area leads to an abnormal sinus cycle. For example, when a sinus opening is obstructed, sinus mucus stagnates and its contents can be altered, leading to damage of the hair cells, with the result of ultimate abnormal drainage. This can lead to a vicious cycle of sinus infection (see Figure 1.4):

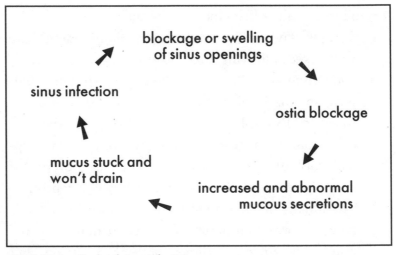

FIGURE 1.4   Cycle of sinus infection.

CONCLUSION

The anatomy and functions of the nose and sinuses are the foundation of understanding how to keep your sinuses healthy. Since many sinus infections start with a common cold, we'll review this malady in Chapter 2. It will offer suggestions for relieving cold symptoms, and for minimizing the chance of developing a sinus infection.

THE COMMON COLD

W hen I wake with a stuffy, runny nose and sore throat, I know that I am usually in for at least four more days of the uncomfortable illness known as the common cold. However, if I were in ancient Greece or China, I would believe that these symptoms should be seen in a positive light. Ancient medicine viewed the cold as a way for the body to clean itself of stored poisons and waste products. Today, we view cold symptoms as a problem, so they will be the focus of this chapter.

Common is an appropriate adjective to describe this viral infection of the nose and the adjacent upper respiratory passages. Colds are by far the most widespread of all infections in this country, affecting more than 150 million people in the United States each year. Many people, especially children, have two or more colds annually. In the average year, colds are responsible for a loss of 440 million workdays and 62 million school days. Including time lost from work, doctors' fees, and medications purchased, the annual cost of colds has been estimated well in excess of eight billion dollars annually.

Sinus infections are often preceded by the common cold. As explained in Chapter 1, a cold causes swelling of the nasal and sinus linings, leading to blockage of the sinus openings, with resultant infection. Once your cold symptoms last more than ten days, you probably have developed a sinus infection. Thus, by understanding how a cold develops, how to obtain relief from cold symptoms, and how to shorten the duration of a cold, you will be able to lessen your risk of sinusitis.

Colds are infections of the lining of the nose. The common cold is caused by a virus—not just a single virus but any one of more than 125. These include rhinovirus, adenovirus, coronavirus, and respiratory syncytial virus. Because so many viral types cause colds, it has been difficult to develop a vaccine that would make you immune to the common cold, since vaccines are targeted at a specific culprit. It also explains why a person who has recovered from one cold is still susceptible to infection by a different virus and thus can catch other colds.

Viruses and bacteria are two different things. Sinus infections are caused by bacteria (bacteria respond to antibiotics), while a cold is secondary to a virus (which does not respond to antibiotics). Patients commonly come in asking for an antibiotic for their cold not realizing that antibiotics will not help them because their cold is caused by a virus. (Later, we'll explain why antibiotics, such as penicillin and the -mycin drugs, may actually be harmful in the treatment of uncomplicated colds.)

The earliest warning that a cold may be developing is often a sensation of dryness or mild irritation at the back of the nose or throat. Sometimes this is felt on the back of the palate in the roof of the mouth. Within twenty-four to thirty-six hours, the nasal passages become stuffy or clogged, and watery discharge develops. Sneezing is often present. The sinuses feel heavy, since swelling of the nasal lining blocks the small openings to the sinuses. The passages that connect the back of the nose to the ears, the eustachian tubes, also swell, often resulting in a sensation of fullness in the ears. A cold is often accompanied by a mild to moderate sore throat (rarely by a severe sore throat, as would be seen with a primary throat infection). There may be a mild cough, as mucus from the back of the nose drips into the lower throat and even into the lung's bronchial tubes. While the cold sufferer may have a mild constitutional reaction, such as generalized aching and fatigue, these symptoms are minimal, with fever, if present, being only mildly elevated.

We catch a cold when a cold sufferer sneezes, coughs, or otherwise transmits the virus to us. A common mode of transmission is the spread of infectious material from hand to hand. This is why children often get colds when they play at local indoor play areas, for example, those with large bins of balls and climbing gyms. You can decrease your child's chance of getting a cold by washing his hands as soon as he is finished playing in one of these "high germ" areas. Similarly, children get frequent colds during school months, since they commonly use their hands and shirtsleeves to wipe their noses, with increased spread of infection. I often see teachers (especially in their first year of work) who have constant upper respiratory infections, as they are in close proximity to these children daily.

Once the virus gets into the upper respiratory passages, it grows rapidly. The nasal lining responds by swelling, as the body increases blood circulation to this region in an effort to fight the infection. Mucus production increases as another of the body's defense mechanisms. Thus, a viral invasion triggers the response that results in the symptoms of a cold. Although most of us were raised to believe that cold weather or sitting in a draft increases susceptibility to a cold, this is not the case. Simply being "cold" will not make you catch cold. Neither does going outside with wet hair.

Although colds can occur throughout the year, they are more frequent at certain times. In temperate climates, rhinoviruses have a seasonal pattern, with fall and spring showing peaks of infection. In the United States, the infection rates for this virus are highest in September. This may be due to the return of children to school, where they are exposed to classmates with respiratory illnesses. This is why anyone with children of school or preschool age will usually have more than their share of colds.

The incubation of rhinovirus infections is two to three days. Viral shedding, or replication, begins a few hours after incubation starts and continues for a week or so. The typical duration of illness in young adults is seven days, but symptoms last up to two weeks in 25 percent of the cases. A cold lasting ten to fourteen days or longer may indicate the development of a bacterial complication, such as a sinus infection. Later in this chapter, we'll get a better idea of how to recognize these complications.

TREATING A COLD

There is no specific or curative treatment for a cold. Yet, many simple measures will provide relief of cold symptoms, and a few readily available medications have been shown to shorten the duration and severity of a cold.

Fluid intake should be increased to twice your normal allotment. This may consist of water, juice, soup, and tea (known as "clear liquids"). Warm liquids seem to be especially soothing. For years we have heard about the healing power of chicken soup. A 1978 scientific study done at Miami's Mt. Sinai Medical Center suggested that chicken soup actually increases mucus flow in the nose, helping to clear out infected material better than other warm liquids. Cutting back on heavy, fatty foods and milk products during a cold may be helpful, since these are felt to increase the production of mucus. However, some studies have shown that milk coats the mouth and throat and may cause the perception of increased mucus, but does not, in fact, increase the actual amount of mucus.

If your cold symptoms are mild, then normal activity and even light exercise is permitted. With a more severe cold, rest can be beneficial. In either case, avoiding fatigue and cutting back on stressful activity is good advice. Smoking, an unhealthy habit anytime, is especially ill-advised during a cold, since it further irritates the lining of the nose and throat, slowing ciliary activity. (You will recall that cilia are the tiny hairs that line the respiratory passages and help to propel the overlying mucus blanket.)

TO BLOW OR NOT TO BLOW?

Many physicians advise their patients not to blow their noses in order to avoid forcing infected secretions at the back of the nose into the eustachian tubes. Nasal congestion and blockage of this tube can set up a possible ear infection. This problem occurs if the patient with a cold presses on both sides of the nose with the handkerchief or tissue when blowing. When I get a cold (yes, doctors are subject to the same maladies as their patients), I feel some relief when thick mucus is cleared by blowing my nose. So I advise patients that they can safely clear secretions from the nose by blowing with one or both nostrils open. There is no better source of reinfection for a respiratory illness than a handkerchief into which the cold sufferer sneezes and coughs all day. Disposable paper tissues are preferred, with a paper bag or trash can close at hand to discard used tissues.

Children often sniff back in order to clear their noses. This habit is distressing to parents, especially when repeated frequently. In reality, sniffing is a safe, effective method of clearing mucus from the nose. Secretions removed in this manner cannot be forced into the eustachian tubes or into the ear channels.

Six-year-old Philip was brought to me by his parents, distressed by his constant sniffing. It had started two months prior following a severe cold and had reached a point that even his kindergarten teacher had brought it to their attention. During his office visit, Philip sniffed and snorted every ten to fifteen seconds. I found no underlying medical problem but did notice that when he was distracted during the examination he did not sniff. Once I explained to his parents that this had become a habit, the symptoms soon subsided as less attention was paid to them.

When a child (like Philip) has nasal congestion for a prolonged period of time, sniffing may become a habit that persists even after the original cause has cleared. Frequently admonishing the child who sniffs only reinforces the habit. Create a well-humidified environment, and wait several days to see if the sniffing clears on its own. If not, then examination by a physician is advised in order to rule out a physical cause for the problem, such as thick secretions in the back of the nose. Most "sniffers" probably have an underlying allergic problem.

CAN A COUGH BE GOOD?

Not only does a cough often accompany a cold, but it also occurs with other respiratory illnesses. Not all coughs are "bad," since the cough itself is a protective reflex that helps clear the windpipe and bronchial tubes of secretions. Medications that suppress a cough can relieve this annoying symptom and permit rest but have no specific effect on the underlying illness. Drinking warm liquids (tea or soup) and sucking on cough drops are helpful. A number of cough medications can be purchased without a prescription (see Chapter 8). Many stronger anti-cough products contain codeine or other prescription drugs. If your cough persists, examination and treatment by a physician is warranted.

HELP NATURE WITH HUMIDITY

Creation of a well-humidified environment is helpful to the patient with a cold, especially when he has an accompanying cough. The lining of the entire respiratory system (nose, throat, and bronchial tubes) is covered by microscopic hairs called cilia. The cilia beat back and forth, clearing out mucus, bacteria, and other material. These cilia operate properly in a moist atmosphere but fail to do so when inhaled air is too dry. Most homes, especially those with hot-air heat, have much lower-than-optimal humidity. By increasing the amount of water vapor in the air, this condition can be remedied. How about opening a bedroom window at night? If the air outside is well humidified, won't this keep your bedroom moist? No, because warm air (inside your house) can hold many times more moisture than cold outside air. For example, 70-degree air can hold more than twenty times as much moisture as 0-degree air. So, cold outdoor air that has a high relative humidity becomes poorly humidified when it is heated indoors.

A humidifier provides relief by putting particles of water into the air and can be used in a room-sized unit or in a larger central unit in the case of a forced hot–air system. A vaporizer converts a liquid (water) into a gas (water vapor) and puts steam into the air. Both the humidifier (cool air) and the vaporizer (steam) work by improving humidity and putting moisture into the air. Humidifiers work by relieving the dry mouth that results when the nose is blocked, and improving ciliary action.

Some people, on the other hand, find the steam of the vaporizer to be more soothing. However, when a vaporizer is used for a child, one must be cautious about having a basin of hot water sitting in the child's bedroom. With cool-air humidifiers, use fresh water each time, and wash the reservoir to prevent fungus growth. Many aromatic products are available for use in a vaporizer, but they have no proven benefits.

COLD MEDICATIONS

Oral Medications

Although pharmacy shelves are filled with scores of non-prescription "cold medications," almost all of them contain a combination of drugs, including a decongestant, an antihistamine, an analgesic, and sometimes a cough suppressant.

Since the primary symptom of a cold is nasal congestion, a *decongestant* taken orally will open the nasal passages by shrinking the lining of the nose. A plain decongestant should suffice for an uncomplicated cold, or try a decongestant–cough medication when coughing accompanies nasal congestion. Plain decongestants available without a prescription include Sudafed tablets, Novahistine DMX, Robitussin PE, and Vick's 44 (a full listing of cold medications and their components is presented in Chapter 8). Do not take decongestants if you have high blood pressure, heart disease, thyroid disease, glaucoma, or difficulty in urination because of an enlarged prostate gland, since decongestants may exacerbate these conditions. In many people, decongestants cause wakefulness, so avoid the evening dose.

Antihistamines have little place in combating this viral illness—the common cold. They fight allergy symptoms and may decrease a runny nose, with their drying effect. However, this drying of nasal secretions thickens mucus in the nose and throat, and may lead to plugging of the sinuses or blockage of the eustachian tubes. Furthermore, most nonprescription antihistamines can cause drowsiness, and should be avoided when driving or working with machinery. I recommend you check your medication to make sure it doesn't have an antihistamine when you don't need one.

Analgesics, such as aspirin or acetaminophen (Tylenol), are useful in relieving pain or reducing fever but have no effect on the nasal symptoms of a cold. *Cough medication* can provide relief of the cough that may accompany a cold.

Nasal Sprays

If you cannot take a decongestant for one of the reasons noted above, a number of *decongestant nasal sprays or drops* can be purchased without a prescription. These include Neo-Synephrine, Afrin, Duration, Dristan, Sine-Off, and Sinex. These medications open the nasal passages by decreasing the swollen nasal lining. Sprays tend to carry the medication to a larger area than do nose drops. The use of nasal sprays such as those listed should be restricted to three or four days, since extended use may result in addiction. As the effect of a spray or drops wears off, the user experiences a "rebound" of the nasal lining, with increased swelling. This results in more-frequent application of the medication, setting up a cycle of reduced effectiveness and rebound congestion. So limit your usage of these products.

Nose sprays and drops have a long and interesting history. As long ago as three thousand years, the Chinese inhaled vapors from a plant called "horsetail" to relieve congestion. We know today that this plant contains the drug ephedrine, which is a decongestant. Another nose drop that was used in the first half of this century was Argyrol, the black nose drops that those older than sixty may remember. While these drops did fight infection, they were also found to have an adverse effect on the hair cells lining the nose, so their use was eventually discontinued.

Vitamin C

The final word on the value of vitamin C in preventing or treating a cold has yet to be written. The late Dr. Linus Pauling, a distinguished scientist and Nobel Prize winner, was one of the first to popularize the use of large doses of vitamin C to prevent disease. Subsequent studies on this subject have been less than conclusive, although some data suggest that this vitamin will diminish the severity of a cold. For people who are prone to colds (three or more in a year), I advise daily intake of 1,000 milligrams of vitamin C. This dosage should be doubled at the onset of a cold.

Since vitamin C in high doses may lead to the development of kidney stones, it should be used cautiously in people with a history of stones. Mild diarrhea has also been reported as a result of large doses of vitamin C.

Can Zinc Zap a Cold?

Zinc is a trace element that plays a role in biological systems. It has been shown to disrupt the replication of some cold-causing viruses. Zinc has a beneficial effect on our immune system (the immune system fights infection). In well-designed clinical studies, zinc gluconate in lozenge form reduces the severity and duration of cold symptoms. If zinc is taken in tablet form, it does not yield the results obtained with lozenges. Side effects of zinc tend to be minor but include objectionable taste and mouth irritation. Some zinc lozenges contain a flavoring to make them more palatable. However, some additives intended to mask the taste of the zinc gluconate may inactivate its beneficial effects. So avoid zinc lozenges that contain citrate, tartrate, sorbitol, or mannitol.

For best results, zinc lozenges, a nonprescription medication found in most pharmacies and health-food stores, should be taken as soon as possible at the onset of a cold. The dosage is two lozenges to start, followed by one every two to three hours while awake. Remember to dissolve the lozenge in the back of your throat, and don't chew or swallow it.

Antibiotics

Many cold sufferers are anxious to have their doctor prescribe antibiotics, such as penicillin, a -mycin drug (such as erythromycin), or even one of the newer broad-spectrum antibiotics. *Antibiotics have no effect on any of the viruses that cause the common cold.* Aside from having no place in treatment of a cold, antibiotics have side effects and add needless cost. A more serious consequence of prescribing antibiotics for a cold and other viral illnesses is that it increases the development of bacterial resistance to antibiotics. For example, several decades ago, penicillin was effective against all streptococcal infections and many staphylococcal infections. Now penicillin rarely kills any staphylococcal bacteria and is losing its effect against certain streptococcal strains.

Antibiotics do have a place in treating the bacterial complications of a cold. Thus, your physician may appropriately prescribe antibiotics if your cold starts to develop into something more, such as an ear infection, sinus infection, or bronchitis. Sometimes a culture test is taken from the nose or throat to determine the presence of bacteria, as with a throat culture for strep throat. This test may also provide your physician with information as to which of the antibiotics the offending bacterial is sensitive. Good medical practice mandates that antibiotics be used appropriately for bacterial infections, and that they not be prescribed for colds or other viral infections.

INTERFERON

A naturally occurring substance called interferon has been gaining attention for the past decade. After you have had a cold, there is a period of immunity for about six weeks. During this time, the body is protected by interferon, a protein material produced as a response to viral illness. Interferon then acts to ward off other viral attacks. It is difficult and expensive to produce in the laboratory, but research scientists are working on a practical method of getting the body to increase its supply of interferon. In addition, studies have shown that intranasally administered interferon has been effective in the prevention of experimentally induced rhinovirus infections. Whether it can help against naturally occurring disease is still being debated.

You may have heard of interferon as a cure for certain forms of cancer. This exciting substance is thought to be able to stimulate the body's defenses against tumors. Unfortunately, only a small amount is available, at a cost of $30,000 to $50,000 to treat one cancer patient. However, it is still in the experimental phase.

HOMEOPATHIC AND NATURAL CURES

Homeopathic remedies have grown popular in recent years; increasingly, they've been used to treat the common cold. Homeopathic products are "all natural" and are found not only in health-food stores but also in drug stores and large pharmacy chains. Homeopathy is a 200-year-old field based on the theory that small doses of a substance can boost the immune system, helping it to fight against colds, as well as other ailments. Use of these more natural, alternative treatments has grown with recent yearly sales of $3.77 billion. Homeopathic drugs used today for upper respiratory infections include Oscillococcinum (derived from duck heart and liver), Kalium bichromicum (from chromium iron ore), and Calcarea carbonica (from the European edible oyster).

These homeopathic remedies typically lack rigorous scientific studies to back up their claims. The Federal Drug Administration (FDA), which regulates medical products in the United States, cannot control these homeopathic drugs because they were grandfathered into the 1938 law that created the regulation of medicines. However, these natural remedies have essentially no side effects and are not believed to be capable of causing any harm. Often, these products appear on pharmacy shelves alongside standard medications, packaged as all-natural in boxes similar to cold, flu, and sinus remedies.

Herbs can additionally be used against the common cold, especially since some of them stimulate the body's immune system. Garlic is both an antibacterial and an antiviral agent, helping to rid the body of "harmful invaders." *Echinacea purpurea* is a wild American herb that is believed to increase the body's white blood cells, which fight infection. Goldenseal is another herb believed to help with colds by strengthening weakened nasal membranes and increasing the liver's ability to filter out infectious wastes. These herbs can be found in pill form in health-food stores. Since natural herb products cannot be patented, companies have little monetary incentive to carry out scientific studies to support their use. However, herbal treatments have persisted for thousands of years and are palatable to individuals seeking a "natural" treatment for their cold symptoms.

MIND OVER MATTER

Aside from the physical contributors to colds already mentioned, emotional stress may bring on a cold more easily in a susceptible person. It has been well documented that individuals under psychic conflicts have a higher frequency of organic illness, including the common cold. Lucy Freeman, author of *Your Mind Can Stop The Common Cold*, maintains that "you need not catch a cold if you are aware of pyschic conflicts that cause it." While an emotionally stable person can still occasionally catch a cold, a positive mental outlook is of prime importance in decreasing the frequency of and minimizing the course of most physical illnesses.

If all else fails, consider a treatment suggested by Sir William Osler, one of the forefathers of American medicine: "Put your hat on the bedpost, get into bed with a good bottle of whiskey, and drink until you see two hats." This may not clear your cold, but somehow your symptoms won't be as bothersome. (Actually, alcoholic beverages cause swelling of the lining of the nose, and should only be taken in modest quantity for their soporific effects, which may make it easier to sleep.)

A COLD VACCINE?

Vaccines work by injecting a substance into the body and allowing the immune system to make antibodies to fight against the specific ailment. Although there has been much work looking into a vaccination for the common cold, we are still far from a practical vaccine. As noted, because many different virus types are responsible for colds, it has been difficult to develop a vaccine against all of them. However, pharmaceutical companies are still actively pursuing this challenge, since colds account for roughly half of the country's school or work sick days.

Self-Treatment of a Cold

- increase fluids
- blow nose properly or sniff
- use a humidifier
- limit your activity
- take cold medications: decongestant pills and sprays, analgesics, vitamin C, zinc

---

COLD COMPLICATIONS

Most colds last for a week, while some take several days to run their course. The suggestions made earlier in this chapter may shorten the duration and severity of a cold. Fortunately, most colds clear without complications. But sometimes what begins as the typical viral nasal infection of a cold progresses to a similar infection of an adjacent area, such as the ears, sinuses, throat, voice box (causing laryngitis), or bronchial tubes (leading to bronchitis or even pneumonia). At this point, the infection often becomes bacterial. If during the course of the cold, you develop a fever higher than 100 degrees fahrenheit, an earache, pressure over the sinuses with thick, discolored nasal mucus, pain at the back of the throat, tender glands in the neck, vocal hoarseness, or an increasing cough productive of thick mucus, you may have a complication that requires seeing a doctor.

CONCLUSION

While most colds run a benign course, some are complicated by affecting the sinuses. At this point, you may need evaluation by a physician and treatment with prescription medications. The next chapter will explain how sinus problems develop, as well as increase your understanding of this common problem.

SINUSITIS

Many patients who come to my office complaining of sinus trouble do not actually have sinus disease. They may simply have a cold, allergies, or an unrelated headache. This confusion is largely due to the frequent misuse of the term in TV commercials for nonprescription (over-the-counter) medications. Nonetheless, true sinus infections are a common problem that require appropriate medication and, at times, surgery. You need to understand how sinusitis differs from a common cold, and what factors may predispose you to sinusitis.

DEFINING SINUSITIS

Since "-itis" means inflammation, sinusitis refers to inflammation of the lining of one or more of the sinuses. Medically speaking, we classify sinus infections according to the sinuses involved. For example, maxillary sinusitis indicates an infection of the maxillary sinus, which is located in the mid-face. We also indicate which side is involved: right maxillary sinusitis, left maxillary sinusitis, or bilateral maxillary sinusitis when both sides are infected. Any number of your sinuses can be inflamed at one time. When all are infected, the term pansinusitis is applied.

Sinusitis is also classified by its duration and frequency: what we refer to as "acute" sinusitis versus "chronic" sinusitis. *Acute sinusitis* lasts less than six to eight weeks, or occurs less than four times a year. *Chronic sinusitis* is a persistent disease of more than eight weeks' duration, or more than four episodes of infection per year. Acute and chronic sinusitis are essentially different diseases with different symptoms and different courses of treatment.

ACUTE SINUSITIS

While many people confuse the symptoms of a cold with having sinus disease, it does make some sense because acute sinusitis is often preceded by having a cold. If your cold symptoms last longer than ten to fourteen days, you are probably developing a sinus infection. Occasionally, sinusitis follows an allergic flare-up. Take, for example, my patient Benson, who every spring and fall begins with his typical allergy symptoms of sneezing and watery eyes, which require a short course of allergy medications for relief. However, during one season, this progressed to severe headaches, thick, yellow drainage and fevers, which only cleared after three weeks of antibiotics for what had become a sinus infection. Sometimes, sinusitis can occur without a prior cold or allergy attack.

Early in the course of an acute sinus attack, there is nasal blockage and congestion, excessive mucus in the nose and throat, sneezing (especially when there is an allergic component), and some malaise and fatigue. If fever is present, it is usually low-grade. The presence of facial pain or headache suggests that a sinus infection is developing. If the symptoms of a common cold last more than a week, you should begin to suspect a sinus infection. Fever may elevate, and mucus in the nose and throat may become thicker and discolored, usually yellow or green. The postnasal drip will cause throat discomfort, occasional hoarseness, and often a cough. Cough from the postnasal drainage of sinusitis tends to be worse in the morning and at night, as mucus trickles into the windpipe or bronchial tubes. Although my four-year-old son, Sam, was unable to tell me about the postnasal drip he was experiencing last fall, I knew he had a sinus infection, since every night he would begin with a wet, productive cough from the phlegm dripping into his throat when he was in bed. Once I gave him an antibiotic for the sinus infection, the cough stopped. With an acute sinus infection, there may be a feeling of ear blockage. Sinus infection may also lead to swelling of the glands (also known as the lymph nodes) in the neck.

Acute sinusitis is often recognized by pain and tenderness of the sinuses or by facial pressure. This facial pain is probably the most bothersome symptom, and usually brings those with a sinus infection to my office for help.

Remember that most people have four sets of sinuses: Maxillary, ethmoid, frontal, and sphenoid. Each sinus—or group of sinuses in the case of the ethmoids—is represented on the right and left side of the head. These tend to cause symptoms of pain in different locations of the face. Maxillary sinusitis causes pain in the mid-face (below the eyes), cheek, or upper teeth. This dental pain may cause confusion; I have even seen patients who had extensive dental work done on their upper teeth for what was really a maxillary sinus infection. Some have even had teeth pulled! More often, however, I see the patient with tooth pain who brings dental X rays showing that he actually has a maxillary sinus infection. Ethmoid sinus infection triggers pain between the eyes, near the bridge of the nose. Frontal sinusitis usually causes forehead pain. Pain behind the eyes or at the back of the head may indicate sphenoid sinusitis. Table 3.1 will help you figure out which sinuses are involved in your infection, based on the location of your symptoms.

CHRONIC SINUSITIS

Sinus infection that persists more than eight weeks is referred to as chronic sinusitis. It may follow an acute sinus infection that fails to clear completely with treatment. Another common situation is a patient who has recurrent bouts of sinusitis. If you have more than four episodes of sinusitis per year, it is termed chronic sinusitis. Additionally, if you seem to have sinus symptoms for many months and even years, this too is chronic sinusitis. People who have chronic sinusitis need further evaluation and treatment in order to avoid future flare-ups and improve their quality of life.

TABLE 3.1   Sinuses Involved in Infection

IF YOU HAVE:	THEN YOU HAVE:
pain between your eyes, if pain is worse with eyeglasses on	*Ethmoid Sinusitis*
pain over your cheekbone, pain like a toothache	*Maxillary Sinusitis*
pain that is severe and over your forehead	*Frontal Sinusitis*
pain that is deep-seated, from many areas, including behind your eyes, at the top of your head, and at the nape of your neck	*Sphenoid Sinusitis*

The most frequent symptom of chronic sinusitis is postnasal drip, with thick mucus in the back of the nose or throat. As it drips into the lower throat onto the vocal cords, or even into the windpipe or bronchial tubes, it may trigger a cough. The resulting cough is most apparent in the morning, when waking, and at night. Thinner, watery postnasal drip may indicate allergies. Postnasal drip may lead to a bad taste in the mouth or bad breath. Dull facial pressure and headache are also common, causing many chronic sinus patients to take daily analgesics, like aspirin or Tylenol.

Another common symptom of chronic sinusitis is nasal congestion or blockage. You may be aware of decreased air passage on one or both sides of your nose. (If you have problems with nasal blockage, it is covered in detail in the next chapter.) Nasal congestion may extend to the eustachian tubes. This results in ear fullness and occasionally impacts hearing. While some people with chronic sinus infections become run-down and fatigued, fever is uncommon. One of my patients was diagnosed with and treated for chronic fatigue syndrome for two years. After I operated on his sinuses and drained them of thickened mucus, which had accumulated over years, he felt renewed energy and no more fatigue.

Symptoms of Sinusitis

- nasal blockage/nasal congestion
- nasal drainage (thick and discolored)
- postnasal drip
- low-grade fever
- facial pain/headache
- cough
- ear fullness/ear clogging
- bad taste/bad breath

THE SINUS HEADACHE

Because of the many advertisements for sinus pills, we have come to assume that most headaches are associated with sinus problems. This is not the case. Sinus headaches usually begin after a person is up and about in the morning, and usually subside by evening. Headaches occurring at night, especially those that awaken the victim, are rarely, if ever, due to sinus infection. Changes in atmospheric pressure and temperature, however, may bring on sinus inflammation with a headache. For example, sinus head-aches often begin after people experience pressure changes on airplane flights. Some individuals report that their sinus headaches begin when the weather changes, for example, before a storm when the humidity is high. My patient Stanley is usually more accurate than the local weather-man at predicting a severe thunderstorm; he calls my office for a renewal of the antibiotic he takes for his sinus headaches, which start when the air humidity is high. (In Chapter 6, we will take an in-depth look at the many causes of headache.)

Headaches or facial pressure associated with sinusitis are often accompanied by some degree of nasal congestion or blockage. If you can relieve sinus pressure by spraying your nose with an over-the-counter decongestant spray (Neo-Synephrine, Afrin) or by taking a decongestant tablet (Sudafed), that suggests that the pressure or headache is sinus in origin. If your headache is stress related, or if it is a migraine, then the decongestants (spray or tablets) will have little effect. Remember that the use of nonprescription decongestant sprays should be limited to three to five days only. Decongestant tablets should not be taken with any regularity by people with high blood pressure or men with prostate problems.

WHAT CAUSES A
SINUS INFECTION TO DEVELOP?

A number of factors predispose one to sinusitis. The most common situation occurs when a viral upper respiratory infection (in other words, a cold) causes swelling and congestion of the lining of the nose. This may result in obstruction of the relatively small sinus openings, decreasing normal sinus ventilation and drainage. That triggers the development of a sinus infection. Sinusitis may begin as a viral infection, but within a few days can progress to a bacterial infection, with pus in the sinus. Pus is a thick material that causes further sinus blockage. This blockage leads to infection, with increased mucus production. This excess of mucus and pus is moved by the cilia that line the sinuses and nose into the back part of the nose, causing the post-nasal drip which accompanies almost all cases of sinusitis.

In many sinus sufferers, especially those with repeated infection, there may be one or more preexisting conditions that contribute to the problem. These include a deviated nasal septum, nasal polyps, or allergies. All of these cause narrowing of the nasal passages, and often blockage of the sinus openings, which increase the chance of a viral cold progressing to a full-blown sinus infection. This is why some people undergo operations such as a deviated septum surgery or nasal polyp removal—to improve their chronic sinus infections. Likewise, I see a number of patients whose sinus infections stopped once they began allergy shots, which addresses the allergic component of their sinus disease.

Several specific conditions trigger sinus infections. I will address these briefly because they are common scenarios that send patients to my office, and thus may be contributing factors in your sinus problems.

DENTAL PROBLEMS

At least several times a year I see a patient with an infected tooth, usually an upper, that leads to infection in the maxillary sinus. Remember that the upper teeth, especially the molars, are located just below the maxillary sinuses (refer to Figure 1.3 on page 5). The bony wall between the roots of the molars and the floor of the maxillary sinus may be quite thin, and an infection that begins in your teeth can travel to the adjacent sinus. This also explains why one of the symptoms of acute maxillary sinusitis can be pain in the upper teeth.

FLYING AND DIVING

Some people get severe sinus attacks following airplane flights or scuba diving because of underlying problems with nasal drainage. When you fly or deep-dive, you experience changes in air pressure. You have probably noticed these pressure changes in your ears during an airplane takeoff. This is because the eustachian tube between your nose and ears functions to equalize these pressure changes so that they won't damage your head and its intricate structures. This is what gives you the ear-popping feeling when driving uphill, riding in an elevator, or flying in an airplane. Pressure changes can cause swelling of the sinus membranes and lead to inflammation and, at times, to infection. If you have a cold, these problems become worse. An easy remedy I give my patients is an oral decongestant like Sudafed to be taken a half hour before the plane takes off (or before scuba diving), and a topical decongestant nasal spray (such as Afrin or Neo-Synephrine) during ascent and descent (and mid-flight for longer trips). The decongestants keep the nasal passages open and help prevent blockage. For infants and young children, who don't know how to clear their ears, give them a bottle or encourage swallowing while the plane is landing.

PREGNANCY

During pregnancy, many women experience "rhinitis of pregnancy" (inflammation of the nose), which is characterized by swelling of the nasal lining, with associated mucus drainage. This condition is due to hormonal changes that occur during pregnancy. Interestingly, individuals who take birth control pills (which cause the body to mimic the hormonal state of pregnancy) may also experience nasal symptoms. As with anything that causes swelling of the nasal membranes, rhinitis of pregnancy may lead to a sinus infection. This can be problematic to treat because there are limitations to medications an expectant mother can take. While most physicians are reluctant to prescribe much medication for pregnant women, the use of a saltwater nasal spray or a nonprescription decongestant spray to open the nasal passages may be acceptable. If infection develops, then an antibiotic may be necessary. If you are pregnant, check with your obstetrician before taking any medication.

IMMUNOSUPPRESSED PATIENTS

As medical treatment becomes more sophisticated, we see an increasing number of patients who are "immunosuppressed," or have poorly functioning immune systems.

These include patients on chemotherapy or radiation therapy, and those who have had organ transplants. AIDS and HIV-positive patients also have weakened immune systems and may be unable to fight the typical sinus infection. Any of these patients should be under close medical care during treatment for sinus infections. If sinus infections are left untreated, serious complications can result, with the infection spreading to nearby structures, including the eye or the brain. Additionally, immunocompromised patients can have unusual types of organisms growing in their sinuses, such as fungus, which can be destructive; these must be treated aggressively.

ASTHMA

Asthma is a disease of lower-lung airway sensitivity to a variety of stimuli. Asthma sufferers are more likely than the average person to have sinus problems. If you have asthma, you may also have hyperactive nasal airways, which lead to sinusitis or nasal polyps. Allergies are also commonly present with asthma and sinusitis, and thus it is felt that the two are interrelated diseases. In addition, patients with asthma may be sensitive to the dripping from a sinus infection. The infected pus that drips from your nose into your throat can exacerbate or set off an asthma attack. It is important for patients with asthma to seek medical attention with early signs of a sinus infection to prevent their asthma from getting worse.

I have a number of asthmatic patients I follow who have chronic sinus complaints. Take for example Amie, a twenty-nine year old who endured asthma for years; she intermittently needed inhalers but had never required oral

41

medications until nine months prior to seeing me. When I questioned her, it became evident that her asthma had worsened after a severe sinus infection over the winter months. After close physical exam and X-ray studies revealed nasal polyps and chronic sinus infection, she underwent surgery on her nose and sinuses and was taken off all her oral pulmonary medications without a problem.

PREVENTING A SINUS INFECTION

Before calling a doctor about your sinus problem, a number of simple things can be done at home. Since the earliest stages of acute sinusitis begin as a viral upper respiratory infection, measures to relieve a common cold (see Chapter 2) may be helpful. Rest, increasing fluid intake, decongestants, and improved humidity will decrease some symptoms. These measures may even lessen the chances of developing acute sinusitis. With the development of pain over one of the sinus locations outlined earlier, or with a rising temperature, prompt evaluation and treatment by a physician is necessary. In addition to the physical examination, your doctor may order X rays of your sinuses or take a culture from your nose. (Your physician's role in your sinus infection is further described in Chapter 9.) Often, prescription antibiotics will be ordered to fight the bacterial infection of sinusitis. Other medications that help ease bothersome symptoms may be recommended, and these are outlined in detail in Chapter 8.

Acute sinusitis may progress rapidly, and on occasion may result in the spread of infection to tissues surrounding the eye or even the lining of the brain. Early treatment of sinusitis by a physician will minimize the chance that acute sinusitis will progress to a serious complication or a chronic sinus infection. A person who has previously experienced an acute sinus infection will usually recognize early on the start of a new episode, and will hopefully seek medical attention as soon as possible.

Some general lifestyle changes can help those with chronic sinus complaints. A well-balanced diet, plus daily vitamin intake (including vitamin C) will help maintain a more normal mucous blanket. Smoke, either primary or secondary exposure, aggravates sinus problems and should be avoided. Likewise, air pollution in general contributes to sinusitis and may explain the rise in sinus disease in recent years in industrialized nations. Steam inhalation is an excellent and relatively harmless way to effectively aid in sinus drainage. Either cool or warm mist is useful, and can be used at the first sign of a sinus infection. If a towel over a basin of hot water doesn't work, you can use a facial cosmetic steamer or a steamer specifically designed for sinus patients. There are a number of commercially available sinus-irrigation systems, and a list of some of these is provided in the references at the end of the book. Over-the-counter medications, specifically decongestants and antihistamines, can decrease annoying symptoms. However, symptoms that persist require evaluation by a physician.

CONCLUSION

Patients who have recurrent or long-standing nasal or sinus symptoms usually have one or more of the following problems: Chronic infections, anatomic nasal obstruction, or allergies. We have already reviewed acute and chronic infections. In Chapter 4 we'll discuss nasal obstruction, and in Chapter 5, allergies.

NASAL OBSTRUCTION

A common complaint of many individuals with sinus problems is a "blocked nose." This feeling of blockage can result from sinus infections. In addition, there are a number of things that anatomically block the nose and can lead to sinus problems. Blockage may occur when the lining of the nose swells, or when there is a deformity of the cartilaginous or bony structures that make up the framework of the nose. This chapter will explore the common conditions that cause nasal blockage and how they can be treated.

NORMAL NASAL BLOCKAGE:
THE NASAL CYCLE

You may notice one side of your nose feeling blocked, and sometime later feel that the other side is clogged. Many people notice this at night when lying in bed, since they have to alternate sides they sleep on to be able to breathe comfortably. This is what is termed the "nasal cycle," which is the normal cycle of congestion (swelling) and decongestion (shrinkage) in the nose. The nasal cycle causes swelling and then shrinkage of the linings of each side of the nose. The blood vessels inside the lining of the nose become engorged in a cyclic fashion, which leads to this swelling and shrinkage.

This cycle varies from person to person but normally takes one to four hours. If you hold a finger over one nostril and blow air out the other nostril, you will notice a different amount of air coming from each side. This should normally vary from side to side according to your nasal cycle. Several factors affect the nasal cycle. For example, if you lie on your side, the nostril that is on top becomes more open. Emotional excitement causes nerves inside the nose to make the lining swell. Thus, you may notice intermittent swelling in your nose and still be within the range of normal.

NASAL SWELLING

Many conditions lead to abnormal swelling of the linings of the nose, causing the sensation of constant blockage. It is important to realize when these factors are contributors to your nasal obstruction. Otherwise, you could undergo surgery to correct what was thought to be a purely anatomic problem yet still be unable to breathe through your nose. If you have already had surgery, for example, straightening of a deviated septum (this will be covered later in the chapter), but still feel that your nose is blocked, perhaps you have one of these underlying problems.

CHRONIC SINUSITIS

One of the most annoying symptoms for people with chronic sinus disease is the feeling of nasal stuffiness. The poor airflow in the nose that results from chronic infection causes nasal blockage, which can be intermittent or constant. When it is constant, it may be the result of an anatomic abnormality. These anatomic blockages can additionally block the "ostia" or openings of the sinuses, leading to recurrent infections. In this way, chronic sinusitis and nasal obstruction are intimately related.

ALLERGIES

An allergy indicates that you are overly sensitive to something in the environment or to certain foods. When you are exposed to something to which you are allergic, it causes a reaction in the nasal lining that leads to swelling. In addition to this symptom of nasal congestion, individuals with allergies experience frequent sneezing, watery eyes, and thin nasal drainage. Allergies can be treated by avoidance, medications or sprays, and for severe cases, allergy shots. (We will discuss allergy in greater detail in the next chapter, since it can be a strong contributor to sinus problems.)

NOSE DROP OR NOSE SPRAY OVERUSE

The medical term for this condition is *rhinitis medicamentosa.* It means nasal stuffiness due to the overuse of decongestant sprays or drops. Decongestant sprays (which are purchased over-the-counter) initially decrease the lining of the nose and give great relief to the congested patient. However, using these sprays for more than a few days leads to a rebound, whereby the lining of the nose becomes even more swollen than before the drops were used. This leads to the addiction, which I see at least weekly in my office, when a patient has used nose drops every day for months or even years yet still feels constant nasal stuffiness. The solution is to stop the decongestant spray completely, so that the swollen nasal lining can return to a normal state. I actually encourage patients with this problem to throw out the spray that caused it so they won't be tempted to continue to use it. To obtain relief during this weaning period, they should take a decongestant tablet (like nonprescription Sudafed) or a short tapering dose of oral cortisone (a prescription drug) to reduce nasal swelling. A saltwater (saline) nasal spray can be used as often as necessary to provide moisture to the irritated nasal lining. Some physicians prescribe a cortisone spray, since these do not induce the rebound phenomenon seen in the "Afrin addict."

BIRTH CONTROL PILLS

Birth control pills have become an increasingly frequent cause for nasal congestion. Take, for example, Perri, a young woman who began to experience severe nasal congestion during her freshman year of college. When I examined her and saw no anatomic problem inside her nose, I asked her questions about her environment. However, she was commuting to school from home and thus had few new exposures. In further discussion, she revealed to have recently begun using birth control pills. Once I had her stop using them, her nasal symptoms subsided.

If your doctor can find no other obvious cause for your nasal stuffiness, or if your symptoms seem coincident with your use of the Pill, then it may be wise to try a two-month period off the Pill to see if your symptoms subside. If they do, then it may be reasonable to seek alternative means of contraception. The hormones in birth control pills cause swelling of the nasal lining. This is similar to the nasal symptoms that some women experience during pregnancy (see Chapter 3), since the purpose of birth control pills is to create a similar hormonal state to pregnancy, and thus avoid conception.

HYPERTENSION

Although hypertension (high blood pressure) itself does not cause nasal blockage, some of the medicines used to treat it, for example, Reserpine, can cause nasal stuffiness. It is best to check with the doctor who prescribes the blood-pressure medicine, and to see if you can switch to an alternative. Decongestants should not be used by hypertensive patients without their doctor's okay, since they can cause blood-pressure elevation.

THYROID PROBLEMS

Hormones are substances excreted in one part of the body but can affect distant locations in the body. For example, the neck's thyroid gland secretes thyroid hormone, which affects metabolism all over the body. One sign of an underactive thyroid is nasal swelling. Other signs of hypothyroidism (low thyroid hormone) include weight gain, fatigue, facial puffiness, and brittle hair. Telling your doctor of these symptoms may help him discern the cause of your nasal blockage. Treatment with thyroid medication should improve the nasal symptoms.

ANATOMIC CAUSES
OF NASAL OBSTRUCTION

Many anatomic factors cause nasal obstruction. You might suspect an anatomic blockage when your breathing always seems worse on one side of the nose, and if the blockage has been present for many months or years. Remember that the two major components of the nasal passages are the septum and the turbinates. Significant abnormalities of these structures will impair breathing. In addition to nasal blockage, they can lead to snoring (which can be disruptive to the individual if he has apnea or pauses in breathing, but is more often a nuisance to a sleeping partner). Additionally, areas that block airflow in the nose can also block mucous flow and sinus drainage, and lead to sinus infections. Much of the remaining portions of this chapter will examine these anatomic causes of nasal obstruction.

DEVIATED SEPTUM

The nasal septum is the partition between the right and left sides of the nose. It is composed of both cartilage and bone. Figure 4.1 shows a normal midline septum compared with a septum that is severely deviated into the right side. A deviated septum is usually diagnosed when a physician looks inside the nose. One clue is to breathe in and out through each side of the nose while blocking the other nostril. A consistent difference in airflow between the two sides may indicate a deviated septum. If you have an obvious twist to the outside of your nose, this may also indicate a deviation on the inside.

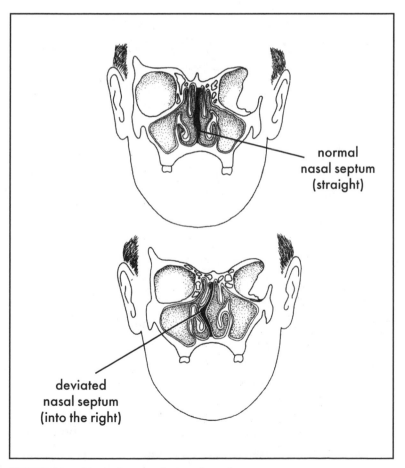

normal
nasal septum
(straight)

deviated
nasal septum
(into the right)

FIGURE 4.1   Normal versus deviated nasal septum.

Often, a deviated septum results from a nasal injury. Some of my patients who have septal deviations remember the exact incident when they fractured or broke their nose, and recall breathing problems beginning after this. Other people are unable to recall any nasal trauma. No one knows whether these individuals were born with their deviation, or whether they suffered some trauma to their developing nose while sliding down the vaginal canal during birth. If the twist of the septum does not seem to harm your breathing, then there is no reason to correct the problem. However, if the deviation is severe enough to warrant repair, you may need surgery. There may also be instances when the septum needs to be fixed not for breathing but because it blocks the sinus openings, leading to chronic sinus infection.

Surgery for a deviated septum involves working inside the nose to reshape the cartilage and bone, either called a septoplasty or submucous resection. It is performed on an outpatient basis under either general ("all the way under") or local (sedation) anesthesia. The septum sometimes needs to be straightened during sinus surgery so that the surgeon can reach back to the sinuses. Correction of a deviated septum usually does not change the outer appearance of the nose. If someone says they had a deviated septum operation but they look like they have a new nose, they are probably covering up elective cosmetic surgery.

HYPERTROPHIC (ENLARGED) TURBINATE BONES

There are three sets of paired turbinates in the nose: inferior, middle, and superior. Refer to Figure 1.3 on page 5.

Inferior Turbinate Problems

Large inferior turbinates can lead to blockage in nasal breathing. While some physicians feel that turbinate swelling has a minimal role in nasal dynamics, others believe it is a major contributor to problems. There is still controversy among physicians as to how often inferior turbinate hypertrophy (the medical term for enlargement) needs to be treated. In addition, there is not even agreement as to the best method of treatment for enlarged turbinate bones. While some doctors will inject turbinate tissue with cortisone to decrease swelling, others believe in surgical cautery, laser, or trimming. It is best to ask your doctor to delineate the pros and cons of this treatment if it has been recommended for you.

Middle Turbinate Problems

Middle turbinates can be abnormally shaped, which can lead to "nasal headaches." In addition, most of the important sinus drainage occurs just below the middle turbinate, and thus abnormal formations of the turbinate can lead to significant sinus problems.

A paradoxically shaped middle turbinate, instead of spiraling outward, curves inward, touching the nasal septum as well as narrowing the area of maxillary sinus drainage. When two structures, such as the septum and the middle turbinate, come into contact, this can set off pain fibers and result in headache. If the already large middle turbinate gets more swollen during an allergy attack, this can further block sinus drainage and cause an infection. Surgical trimming of the turbinate should correct the problem.

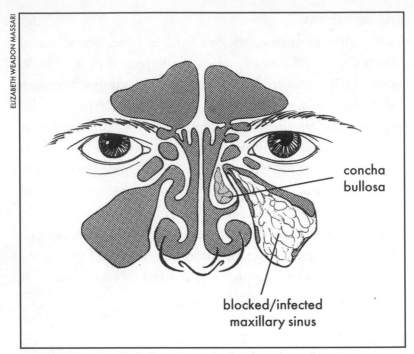

concha
bullosa

blocked/infected
maxillary sinus

FIGURE 4.2   Concha bullosa. Secondarily infected maxillary sinus.

Normally, the turbinates are bony structures lined with nasal mucosa. If developmentally, the middle turbinate has air inside it (which is seen in Figure 4.2), sinus drainage can be altered and may result in recurrent infection.

This condition, in which there is an air cell inside the normally bony middle turbinate, is termed a *concha bullosa* and may additionally be associated with headache. If you have a concha bullosa, then the sinus problem may be alleviated by surgically opening up this air pocket inside the turbinate; this should lead to improved sinus drainage.

Last year, Betsy came to see me after she had gone to an allergist, neurologist, and chiropractor for facial headaches. Because of some underlying nasal complaints, I ordered a CAT scan X ray, which revealed a middle turbinate with air inside (the concha bullosa). I had Betsy come to my office during one of her headaches, and I injected her middle turbinate with a local anesthetic, after which her headache resolved. I next took her to the operating room, where I removed her middle turbinate. She has not had a headache since!

NASAL POLYPS

Polyps are grapelike, inflammatory swellings of the nasal and sinus linings. Polyps are benign (noncancerous), can be on one or both sides of the nose, and are more commonly seen in adults than in children. By far, the most common cause of polyps is allergy, followed by chronic sinus infection. Aside from causing nasal blockage, polyps may plug up the normal sinus openings (ostia) and contribute to the development of sinus infection. While nasal polyps in children are atypical, their occurrence before age sixteen may indicate cystic fibrosis. (See Chapter 7 for more on this childhood disease.)

Nasal polyps may be associated with asthma. I often see an asthma patient whose asthma has flared up because of nasal polyps and sinus infection. Scott is one of my typical asthma patients with nasal polyps. When he first came to see me, he was on a number of asthma inhalers and for the past four months had been using oral medications for worsening symptoms. Once I removed his massive nasal polyps, his breathing greatly improved, and he stopped taking the meds. About once a year Scott will see me complaining of a flare-up of his asthma, when his nose and sinuses act up. I give him some oral cortisone, which shrinks the polyps, and he is back to normal.

In some patients, there is an association between asthma, nasal polyps, and aspirin intolerance known as Samter's triad. Almost one out of four patients with nasal polyps has an intolerance to aspirin. In these people, ingestion of aspirin is followed by wheezing, excessive watery nasal discharge, and swelling of the throat, which can be fatal if not treated immediately.

The initial treatment of nasal polyps is usually medical. Polyps shrink after a course of cortisone (or other steroid) pills, but few patients are kept on this medication for more than several weeks because of potential side effects. If there is significant shrinkage following the taking of cortisone tablets, then an extended course of a cortisone-containing nasal spray may keep the nasal passages clear and prevent reformation of polyps. Cortisone-containing sprays have rare, minor side effects, so they can be used safely in most people for many months under a doctor's supervision. They do not cause rebound congestion as is seen with nonprescription decongestant sprays.

Despite appropriate medication, many polyp patients require surgery to remove the polyps and open the nasal passages. Surgical polyp removal, or polypectomy, can be performed in an office or outpatient setting. It can be done under either local or general anesthesia, and can be combined with other nasal and sinus surgery. Although most polyps are not cancerous, once removed, they are sent for pathologic examination under a microscope to ensure that there is no malignancy (cancer) present. While most patients notice marked improvement in their breathing after removal of polyps, they should be aware that polyps often recur. If they start to grow back in a matter of months, then a more thorough search for the cause should be under-

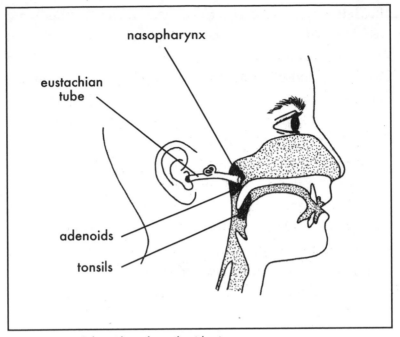

nasopharynx

eustachian
tube

adenoids

tonsils

FIGURE 4.3   Adenoids and tonsils, side view.

taken. This usually includes an allergy workup and CAT scan X ray if they haven't already been done. One way to prevent polyp regrowth after removal is to stay on topical steroid sprays for an extended period of time.

In general, polyps can be a nuisance but are rarely life-threatening. However, certain types of polyps have a predisposition to turn into cancer, and thus if you have polyps, it is best to have a physician fully evaluate them.

ENLARGED ADENOIDS

Adenoid tissue sits at the back of the nose in an area called the nasopharynx (see Figure 4.3). This tissue is similar to tonsil tissue, which is located on each side of the throat. The adenoids shrink and usually become insignificant by the late teens or early twenties. However, there are instances when this tissue remains enlarged in an adult and may be chronically infected; that causes bilateral (both sides of the nose) nasal obstruction. These large adenoids can also contribute to sinus infection. Whenever the adenoids are significantly enlarged in an adult, one must always be concerned about a possible tumor, and thus your doctor may recommend adenoid removal to obtain a biopsy of the tissue for lab evaluation.

The adenoids tend to play a more central role in sinusitis in children, and this is covered in greater detail in Chapter 7. I have many pediatric patients who have been diagnosed with recurrent episodes of sinusitis. Once their adenoids are surgically removed (known as an adenoidectomy), their sinus problems often vanish.

FOREIGN BODY IN THE NOSE

Every so often I see a patient like Ellen, a three-year-old girl whose pediatrician sent her in for what she thought was a sinus infection. The little girl had already been on four weeks of antibiotics but persisted with thick, yellow drainage from her right nostril. Upon close inspection, I found a small bead embedded in the right side of Ellen's nose. Once it was removed, her nasal drainage stopped. Foreign bodies should be suspected in an individual with one-sided nasal drainage. Typically, foreign objects in the nose occur in children or in mentally retarded individuals. Among the things that I have retrieved from inside the nose include buttons, crayons, small plastic toys, peanuts, raisins, popcorn, and pencil erasers.

Causes of Nasal Obstruction

NONANATOMIC

- chronic sinusitis
- allergies
- overuse of nose sprays
- birth control pills
- hypertension
- thyroid abnormality

ANATOMIC

- deviated septum
- nasal polyps
- large adenoids
- nasal foreign body
- hypertrophic turbinate bones

CONCLUSION

Nasal obstruction is a common symptom seen in sinus disease. Additionally, nasal obstruction can lead to blockage of sinus openings, and cause sinusitis. We have covered some of the more common causes of nasal obstuction. As mentioned, allergy is another source of blockage and a prevalent problem in sinus patients. The next chapter will examine allergy in more detail, with attention to diagnosis and treatment.

THE ALLERGIC COMPONENT

Allergies can often be confused with sinus problems. Every spring, when the pollen count rises, I see a number of patients like Gwen, a mother of two, who began her visit by telling me that her "sinuses were acting up again." When I questioned her about her symptoms, she described nasal congestion, itchy eyes, scratchy throat, sneezing, and thin nasal drainage, all causing her to go through a box of tissues every two days. Medications aimed at treating allergies immediately gave her relief from what was actually not sinus disease but classic allergy.

As you can see, allergies are different from sinus disease, although they may be a major contributor leading to sinus infections. This chapter will explore the fundamentals of allergy, including diagnosis and treatment, since attacking the allergy component of your sinus disease can often alleviate much of your nasal problem.

DEFINING ALLERGIES

Allergy is derived from the Greek words meaning "other action," implying a hypersensitivity to a specific sub-stance(s) that does not cause symptoms in most people. Certain substances, called allergens, trigger an allergic response in susceptible individuals. They can enter the body via inhalation, ingestion, injection, and external skin contact. These allergens react with antibodies (certain mole-cules in the immune system) in the allergic person, causing the production of histamine and other chemical substances that cause various symptoms, which we will describe in detail later in this chapter. Thus begins a chain reaction known as the allergic response (see Figure 5.1).

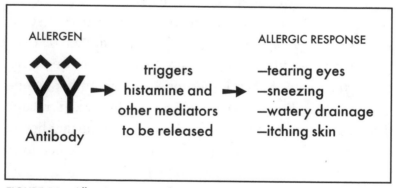

FIGURE 5.1   Allergic response chain reaction.

For example, you may be allergic to pollen. During certain seasons, when the pollen count is high, exposure to pollen (the allergen) sparks an allergic response in your body. This causes histamine release, which leads to sneezing, watery nasal drainage, tearing eyes, and other symptoms we know as allergy.

When an allergen triggers this allergic response, a variety of symptoms can occur throughout the body. While we will concentrate on the nasal aspects of allergy, other systems are also affected, including the skin (with eczema and itching), and the gastrointestinal tract (with heartburn).

Allergy Symptoms

- sneezing
- itching
- nasal drainage (thin, clear, watery)
- nasal stuffiness
- tearing, watery eyes
- "allergic shiners" around eyes
- irritability, fatigue

The nasal symptoms of allergy are termed *allergic rhinitis.* Prominent nasal manifestations include congestion of the nasal membranes, sneezing, and itching. Swelling of the nasal lining leads to the sensation of blockage and possibly to headaches. The nasal drainage in allergic patients is usually thin and clear (as opposed to the thick, colored mucus of infections). In adults, this can lead to watery postnasal drip and cough. In children, the itching nose with thin drainage leads to frequent rubbing upward of the nasal tip called the "allergic salute." Itchy, watery eyes may accompany these nasal symptoms. There may be puffiness and discoloration around the eyes which is termed *allergic shiners* (black eyes of allergy). When allergy symptoms become constant, they may lead to irritability and fatigue.

Nasal allergies tend to run in families, with the allergic individual often having an allergic parent, sibling, or close relative. If one parent is allergic, the child has a 30 to 50 percent chance of inheriting the problem; if both parents have allergies, their children have a 70 percent chance of allergy problems. Some believe that an individual may develop allergies if he has had overstimulation of certain immunoglobulins (which the body produces to help fight infections) by excessive exposure to a certain allergen. For example, some people feel that it may help to withhold common allergy-producing foods until a child's digestive tract is more fully developed in order to decrease food allergies in children. Europeans who have traveled to the United States, where they are exposed to pollen from ragweed (which does not grow in Europe), often develop an allergic response to pollen that is not seen in Europeans who have not traveled.

COMMON ALLERGIES

A number of substances called allergens trigger the allergic response in susceptible individuals. And there are a number of categories of allergens:

Environmental factors are widespread causes of allergy. Most are termed inhalant allergies and are due to substances we breathe. These microscopic particles in the air can lead to a full-blown allergic response. Commonly, these environmental allergies produce symptoms during particular seasons of the year, and are termed *seasonal aller-gies.* When nasal symptoms occur each year during a specific season, one should look for an allergy source. While trees pollinate in the spring and cause springtime symptoms, grasses are important in late spring/early summer allergies, and weeds (such as ragweed) lead to late summer/early fall symptoms. *Perennial allergies,* on the other hand, occur throughout the year. Examples of perennial allergies are mold and dust, found indoors yearlong. There may be clues to such allergies. For instance, house dust may exacerbate symptoms in late fall, when your hot-air furnace is turned on. Other environmental clues are allergies to cats and dogs, seen after exposure to these household pets. Allergy symptoms that are made worse in bed each night may be caused by allergies to pillow feathers.

An exaggerated response to specific food allergens is termed *food allergy* or hypersensitivity. People may crave food to which they are allergic. Although any food may be a cause of allergy, common culprits include milk, eggs, wheat, chocolate, nuts, corn, citrus fruits, pork, and beef.

Medications are also causes of allergy, with rash and itching typically seen. However, these usually don't cause nasal allergic symptoms and will not be considered further in this chapter.

Anaphylaxis refers to those allergic reactions that occur immediately and progress rapidly. These could be life-threatening, as they cause a severe drop in blood pressure or airway narrowing. Examples of anaphylactic reactions include beestings, severe medication reactions, and reactions to ingested food. If you have suffered from an anaphylactic reaction in the past, then you should carry around an injectable shot of a medication called epinephrine, which can be given in an emergency to open up your airway. Clues to identifying some common allergies are outlined in Table 5.1.

TABLE 5.1   Common Allergy Clues

TRIGGER	ALLERGY
May	*grass pollen*
August, September	*ragweed pollen*
late fall, when your hot-air furnace is on	*dust*
in bed each night	*feathers in the pillow*
pet exposure	*dog, cat*

ALLERGIES AND THEIR RELATION TO SINUS DISEASE

As we discussed in earlier chapters, sinus infections occur when there is blockage at the openings (ostia) of normal sinus drainage. One factor that can lead to ostia blockage is allergies. When an individual's allergies are triggered, there is swelling of the nasal linings, which results in sinus blockage and infection. If you seem to get sinus infections during the same time each year, there may be a component of seasonal allergy.

Additionally, polyps, as discussed in Chapter 4, which can underlie sinus disease, are associated with allergy. The incidence of allergy in nasal polyp patients has been found to be up to 60 percent, although the cause-and-effect aspect of this is not fully understood.

While not all patients with chronic sinus disease or nasal polyps need intense allergy evaluation, if symptoms occur, with allergic rhinitis (thin, watery drainage with sneezing, etc.), then allergy factors need to be considered. Table 5.2 should help you discern if your nasal symptoms are infection-related or if they are caused by allergies.

TABLE 5.2   Sinus Infection or Allergy?

INFECTION	ALLERGY
nasal obstruction and congestion	nasal obstruction and congestion
thick nasal discharge	thin, watery nasal discharge
facial pressure and pain	itchy, runny nose
wet, productive cough	dry cough
low-grade fever	sneezing, watery eyes

ALLERGY-TESTING

If your nasal symptoms are not just blockage and infection but consist of sneezing, watery drainage, and other symptoms outlined earlier in this chapter, then you may indeed have allergies. A strong family history of allergy and allergy-related diseases is important to assess. If I suspect an allergy problem in one of my patients, I ask about allergy-related problems in parents, siblings, or children of the patient. Many disorders commonly seen in patients with allergy can be a clue to diagnosis of the underlying problem. These include eczema, asthma, and a variety of gastrointestinal disorders (heartburn, diarrhea, and bloating). Reactions occurring with regularity each year may be due to seasonal allergies, while those that manifest throughout the year are perennial and may be due to household animal dander, dust and mold found indoors, or may possibly represent food sensitivity.

If your symptoms improve with allergy medications (which will be discussed later in the chapter), then you likely have an allergic component to your problems. There are also a variety of tests (which we will discuss) that aid in diagnosis of allergies, helping to discern if your nasal and sinus symptoms may be allergy-related.

Many people wonder if they need to be tested for allergy. I tell my patients to get a test only if it will change their treatment. If you have mild hay-fever symptoms for a few weeks each year, and you respond well to medications, then there is probably no reason to undergo sophisticated allergy-testing. However, if you have nasal congestion with thin, watery drainage yearlong, testing may be helpful in identifying specific factors triggering your allergies. Additionally, if the source of your nasal symptoms is uncertain, allergy-testing may help evaluate the role allergies play in the problem. Below are outlined the more common ways that allergies are tested today.

IN-VIVO TESTING

There are several different ways to test for allergies. One category of test is termed in vivo, meaning "in the living." The basic principle here is to demonstrate an actual allergic reaction in the patient. Various allergens are placed into the skin by either a scratch, a prick, or an injection, and the skin is monitored for a reaction. A "positive" response can be noted when redness or swelling occurs at the injection or scratch site. While these tests can accurately identify actual allergic sensitivities, there is the remote risk of triggering a full-blown allergic response. Another requirement of in-vivo testing is that the patient must stay off his allergy medication for several days prior to testing so as not to invalidate the response. Additionally, this involves the timely and sometimes painful process of injecting numerous allergens, usually on the back or the arms. Skin tests are typically difficult to perform on unwilling infants and young children. Allergic individuals who have skin rashes or hypersensitive skin—which might interfere with test results—are not good candidates for skin testing.

IN-VITRO TESTING

In-vitro testing is based on identifying the antibody proteins produced by the allergic individual during an allergic reaction. A blood sample is collected from the patient, and with sophisticated equipment, the amount of specific antibodies present is measured (there are a variety of antibodies, each of which reacts to a specific allergen). This is called a RAST test, standing for the high-tech testing and machinery (radioallergosorbent test). The RAST test needs only a sample of the patient's blood on which to run the allergy tests. Blood serum can then be run against common allergens, such as dust, mold, pollen, etc.

While the RAST test, with collection of a single test tube of blood, is easy to carry out, it does not verify the actual allergic response in the individual. However, RAST testing is useful in infants and young children unable to be skin-tested, in individuals with extensive skin rashes or skin hypersensitivity, and during the height of the pollen allergy season, since injection may stimulate an overresponse.

NASAL SMEAR

Your doctor may do a nasal smear. Here, a sample of nasal secretions is collected and analyzed in a laboratory. Certain substances (called eosinophils) are produced during an allergic reaction, and these are looked for under a microscope in the nasal specimens obtained. This test does not tell your doctor the specific things to which you are allergic but gives him an idea if your nasal problems are due to allergy.

FOOD DIARY

Another way to identify allergies—specifically food allergies—is to keep a diary of all foods ingested. The diary should include amounts of each food, specific ingredients of everything ingested, and the patient's symptoms. This needs to be recorded for at least a week to offer any meaningful information. The diary can help to target the specific offending agent that causes any allergic symptom.

TREATING YOUR ALLERGIES

ALLERGY PREVENTION

The best way to avoid symptoms of nasal allergy is prevention. This means avoiding exposure to agents that trigger the allergic response. Being aware of common allergens (things that cause allergy) will enable you to minimize your exposure to them. The following suggestions will not apply to every allergic individual, but you can judge which items apply in your case.

Dust is by far the most common inhalant allergy. Creation of a dust-free house is not practical, but developing a dust-free bedroom is important since this is where most allergy exposure occurs. It is also the room where most people spend seven or eight hours each day.

The primary sources of dust in the bedroom are the bed's mattress and box springs. They should be encased in allergy-proof covers. Zippered plastic covers are acceptable if tape is placed over the zippers. Feather or down-filled pillows should be avoided, since both are common allergens. This is also true of foam-rubber pillows, which may grow mold after several years of use. Dacron or other synthetic pillows are recommended for the allergic patient, and a similar pillow should be used by the spouse or roommate.

All stuffed animals, fabric toys, stuffed furniture, and fuzzy blankets should be removed, since these are all dust collectors. No pennants or wall pictures are permitted. Books on bookshelves are dust catchers and should be kept to a minimum. Drapes should be replaced with washable cotton or fiberglass curtains. Venetian blinds are dust collectors and should be avoided. Closet doors should be kept closed, and wool clothing should be placed in plastic bags. Since rugs catch and hold dust, bare wood floors or linoleum are best in the dust-free bedroom. The dust-allergic patient can also prevent allergy attacks by wearing a mask when working in dusty places, making up beds, and emptying the vacuum.

Forced hot–air heating systems are notorious for

circulating dust, but this dust circulation can be reduced with frequent changing or cleaning of the filter and with the use of damp cheesecloth over room air vents. When dust allergy continues to be a problem, you can install an electrostatic air filter adjacent to the central hot-air blower (sometimes this can be a legitimate tax deduction, with a physician's note). An electric heater is much preferred to the hot-air system in allergic households. If a hot-air system already exists, then it should be closed to the allergic person's bedroom and an electric strip heater installed.

If you have seasonal *pollen* and underlying pollen allergies, you will recognize your symptoms during the same season each year. For example, in the eastern United States, grass and tree pollens predominate from April to June; ragweed is common from mid-August to early October. In other sections of the country, different plants cause symptoms during different seasons. Plants that are wind-pollinated produce large amounts of lightweight pollen that can be carried hundreds of miles, triggering an allergic response in susceptible individuals. On the other hand, flower-bearing plants are insect-pollinated, producing heavier, stickier pollen that usually doesn't cause an allergic reaction. If possible, try to avoid exposure to plants that will cause problems.

If you are sensitive to pollen, you should avoid cutting grass, weeding, and exposure to wooded areas. If you must do these gardening chores, wear a filter mask and eyeglasses. When it's your allergy season, spend as much time as possible in an air-conditioned house or car (remember to keep the windows of your house and car closed). Don't bring dried-flower arrangements inside. Since the seashore and mountain areas tend to be pollen-free, you may want to plan a vacation there during the height of pollen season at home. To get an idea of how your symptoms may be each day, you can get the daily pollen count through the National Allergy Bureau's Pollen Count Information Line (800-9-POLLEN) or Website (http:/www.execpc.com/~edi/nab/nab.html). Your local news may also provide the level of pollen in the air in your area.

Mold is a fungus that commonly causes inhalant allergies. There are many varieties of mold, both indoor and outdoor. Molds flourish in cold, damp areas, especially in basements or storage areas. Stuffed furniture is often loaded with mold. While stuffed animals can be a source of mold, if you put them in the dryer for twenty minutes, the heat will kill most of the mold. Barns, dried leaves, cut grass, and dead vegetations are sources of mold. Mold can be minimized with the use of electric dehumidifiers. As a reminder, humidifiers and cool-air vaporizers, which are intended to relieve allergy symptoms, may actually be a source of mold if not regularly cleaned.

Tobacco and *smoke* can trigger a strong allergic response in some individuals. These people should avoid smoking themselves, as well as avoid secondhand smoke. Other sources of allergy include *mothballs, insect spray,* and *fresh paint.* If symptoms grow worse during the Christmas season, when a Christmas *tree* is brought into the house, try an artificial tree. Nasal congestion during swimming may be caused by a *chlorine* allergy.

Avoidance in patients with *food allergies* is somewhat more complex. You may first want to eliminate processed food, since the mere avoidance of chemical additives, sugars, salts, yeast, soy, and spices may be enough to curb allergy symptoms. You may need to ask your doctor about a food-rotation diet, which is designed to prevent sensitization to certain foods.

Breast-fed infants are much less likely to develop allergies than those who receive cow's milk. Breast-feeding should be considered if there is a strong family history of allergy. If this is not feasible, then with your pediatrician's permission, try an allergy-free, soybean or goat's milk.

Animals are another frequent source of allergies. While most of my patient's refuse to give up their dog, cat, or bird (these are the most common allergy-causing animals), some people will agree to keep the animal out of the living or sleeping quarters, or perhaps get a different pet. If you feel that you cannot live without a dog, then your best bet is a poodle, which is considered less of an allergic threat than dogs that shed hair freely. Fish are probably the best pet for the allergic child, since they have no fur or feathers.

ALLERGY MEDICATIONS

If your allergies occur sporadically or for short, seasonal periods, medications may likely provide enough relief. Since the body's allergic reaction is caused by histamine, which triggers the full-blown allergic reaction, medications called *antihistamines* are specific against allergies. They block histamine's activity and prevent its effects on the body. Over-the-counter antihistamines, which will be discussed in greater detail in Chapter 8, include Benadryl, Tavist, Chlor-Trimeton, Dimetane, and Actifed. Their most common side effect is drowsiness, so they should be avoided if you are driving a distance or operating machinery. Antihistamines, while acting to dry up the allergic nasal drip, may lead to excessive dryness of the nose and throat, often bothersome in older patients, who tend to have dry mucosa already. Antihistamines may dry up and thicken the mucus of sinusitis, and thus should only be used in sinus patients with a strong allergic component.

Less frequent side effects of antihistamines include blurred vision, nausea, and confusion. In recent years, some antihistamines have been designed to be "non-sedating," so they don't make you tired. These require a physician's prescription and include Allegra, Claritin, Hismanal, Seldane, and Zyrtec.

In the past few months, an antihistamine in the form of a nasal spray has been introduced into the United States. This prescription spray, called Astelin, works relatively rapidly once sprayed into the nose. The benefit of an antihistamine spray is that it can avoid the unpleasant side effects of oral antihistamines, which impact the entire body.

Combination antihistamine-decongestants are useful in allergic patients who have a strong degree of nasal congestion. While the antihistamine component minimizes sneezing and dripping, the decongestant shrinks the lining of the nose, with resultant improvement in breathing. The decongestant component tends to cause an increasing wakefulness, which counteracts the sedating aspects of antihistamines. Combination antihistamine-decongestants include over-the-counter Allerest, Novahistine, Ornade, and Triaminic, as well as prescription Claritin D (the "D" stands for decongestant), Seldane D, and Semprex. (See Chapter 8 for a more complete list.)

Other combination antihistamine medications may contain additional ingredients such as aspirin and cough suppressants, although these are usually unnecessary for most allergy patients.

Steroids are the most potent medications for the allergic patient, and are available by prescription only. They improve allergies by decreasing the inflammation seen in the allergic reaction. They can be used for a severe flare-up of nasal symptoms, such as during a high pollen season, or when an antihistamine is not strong enough. Continued use of steroids can have serious side effects, so they should be taken on a limited, short-term basis to provide relief and safety. Steroids are available most commonly as cortisone, Medrol, or Prednisone orally, but in severe cases can be given as a shot into a muscle or directly injected into the nose.

Steroids can also be given as a nasal spray, known as an *intranasal steroid spray.* Again, this requires a doctor's prescription. These sprays include Beconase, Flonase, Nasacort, Nasarel, Rhinocort, Nasonex, and Vancenase and work locally on the nasal lining to decrease allergic symptoms of swelling and discharge. They are relatively safe, since they are sprayed directly into the nose and are not absorbed into the bloodstream to give other side effects. Unlike decongestant sprays and drops, steroid nose sprays do not cause a rebound of increased nasal congestion after their use.

Another type of intranasal spray used specifically for allergy symptoms is *cromolyn sodium* (Nasalcrom spray). Cromolyn seems to work by preventing the release of histamine, which causes allergy symptoms. It is most effective if used prior to allergen exposure. For example, if you are allergic to ragweed, it is best to start using Nasalcrom several days before ragweed season begins.

Recently, there has been a spray introduced in the United States called *ipatropium* (known as Atrovent .03 percent and .06 percent). This works differently from other products in that it acts directly on the glands of the nasal lining to decrease the watery drainage that occurs with allergies and other conditions. The higher .06 percent spray is also useful in the common cold when there are excessive amounts of drainage.

ALLERGY SHOTS

If environmental controls and medications have failed to provide adequate relief of allergy symptoms, then the next step of treatment is allergy shots (medically known as allergen immunotherapy or desensitization). Shots are more useful for year-round allergies rather than those lasting a short period each year. There are several methods to allergy shots, but the basic idea is to inject increasing doses of allergens into the allergic patient to sensitize him. The shot is made up of an extract based on results of skin or a RAST allergy test (see earlier in chapter on allergy-testing). Typically, shots are given once to twice every week, with dosage increases with each injection. Sometimes a physician or nurse will give the injection, while other times an extract will be made so that the patient can self-administer it at home. Once a maintenance level is reached, the shots can be given slightly less frequently. Significant improvement should be seen within three to six months of initiating immunotherapy. If successful, the shot should be given for two to five years, at which time the patient should be free of symptoms. When considering allergy shots, it is important that you have tried all other forms of treatment (medications, sprays), since shots require a great deal of commitment and patience before seeing results.

ALLERGY TREATMENT

- Avoidance/prevention

- Medications : antihistamine +/– decongestant
  steroids (oral, nasal)
  cromolyn sodium
  ipratropium

- Desensitization/shots/injections

CONCLUSION

After completing this chapter, you should have a better understanding of allergies: what they are, how they are related to sinus disease, and how they can be treated. We will next turn our attention to headache, which, like allergy, is closely related to and often confused with sinus problems.

HEADACHE

Headache is a frequent symptom of sinusitis, and often the one that brings a patient to my office for treatment. Take, for example, my patient Larry, a company president who flew across the country at least once a week for business. He was plagued by frequent sinus headaches coincident with air flight. Despite long-term antibiotics, decongestants, and nasal sprays, he had persistent pain around the left side of his face and around his left eye. A CAT scan X ray revealed a severe left-sided nasal septal deviation with narrow areas of sinus drainage and inflammation in the left maxillary sinus (cheek) and the left ethmoid sinus (around the eye). After surgery to correct the deviated septum and to widen his sinus openings, he was free of headaches.

There are some patients who, like Larry, have actual "sinus headaches" that respond favorably to treatment of the sinus disease. In fact, most patients who come to me with a history of headaches claim to have "sinus trouble." In reality, only a minority of these individuals actually has headaches that are nasal or sinus in origin. However, most patients with chronic sinus infections do have some degree of headache or facial pain, which must be addressed. It is important to try to differentiate if your headache is sinus in origin or due to another cause, since treatment for different types of headaches varies greatly. Any discussion of sinus disease would be incomplete without the common causes and treatments of headaches, and thus this chapter will explore both the sinus and the non-sinus headache.

THE TRUE SINUS HEADACHE

An acute sinus infection may be accompanied by a headache. In these patients, a common cold or nasal allergy progresses to increasing congestion, fever, and pain in the area of the involved sinus. This headache increases in severity when coughing or bending over. The pain tends to be dull rather than piercing or knifelike. I often find that patients are not bothered by their nasal symptoms as much as by their headaches and facial pain.

As we have discussed earlier, adults have four pairs of sinuses. The frontal sinuses are located over the eyes, with pain presenting in the forehead when these sinuses are infected. Infection of the ethmoid sinuses, located in the deeper recesses of the nose rather than in the front of the face, causes pain between and behind the eyes. The deepest pair of sinuses, named the sphenoid sinuses, results in pain referred to the back of the head. This is a rare occurrence. The maxillary sinuses are located in the middle third of the face, below the eyes and to the side of the nose. These are the most frequently infected sinuses, with pain across the face or in the upper teeth on the affected side.

You should begin to suspect that you have an acute infection of the sinuses when a headache develops in the course of what seems to be only a cold. Acute sinusitis requires treatment by a physician, and usually includes an antibiotic and a decongestant.

Headache may also be a feature of chronic sinusitis. Usually characterized as a dull ache or feeling of fullness, this pressure starts after an individual is up and about in the morning, then lasts until late in the afternoon. It is triggered when congestion of the nasal lining results in contact between adjacent structures in the nose and sinuses. This leads to closing off of a normally patent sinus opening (ostium). When the opening to a sinus is blocked, the air within the sinus is absorbed and cannot be replaced because of the blockage. This results in a negative pressure within the sinus compared with the outside barometric pressure. This pressure, plus any accumulated secretions within the sinus, accounts for sinus headaches. Diagnosis usually requires examination and an X-ray study of the sinuses.

Many common things cause changes in air pressure, with resultant sinus swelling and possible headache. Going up and down in an airplane subjects you to quick changes in atmospheric pressure. This is why flying can lead to sinus (or even ear) trouble in the predisposed individual— one who has an underlying anatomic narrowing. Even if you typically have no problems when flying, if you have an upper respiratory infection and decide to fly anyway, you may end up with a full-blown sinus infection because of the combination of nasal swelling from your cold and pressure changes in the airplane. Taking both an oral and a topical decongestant before takeoff may ameliorate this problem. Scuba diving, with its increased pressure underwater, can similarly lead to sinus swelling and infection.

Another common sinus headache patient I see is typified by Allen, a computer programmer who was debilitated whenever there was a drastic change in the weather. It reached the point where he was better at predicting the forecast than the local TV weatherman. While some might think Allen is crazy, this phenomenon actually has a scientific basis: With changes in atmospheric humidity, pressure changes within the sinuses can cause infection and headache.

CAUSES FOR NON-SINUS HEADACHES

HIGH BLOOD PRESSURE

Headaches may be among the first symptoms of hypertension, or high blood pressure. This headache is often located at the back of the head and is usually noted upon arising in the morning. The pain is throbbing or pulsating. This headache is worsened by exercise, straining, or stooping, since these activities raise blood pressure. A diagnosis can usually be made by checking the blood pressure, which is measured as two numbers: The systolic pressure is listed above the diastolic pressure. A normal reading might be 120/80 (systolic/diastolic). The number 120 (millimeters of mercury) is the systolic pressure, which may vary with activity, exertion, or nervousness. In the diagnosis of hypertension, the diastolic number (in this example 80) is especially important. A diastolic pressure exceeding 100–110 mm (millimeters) of mercury is usually present if hypertension is the true cause of the current headaches. For most patients, treatment consists of medication to lower the pressure, and a low-salt diet and weight reduction when indicated. Evaluation and treatment for high blood pressure are by an internist, family physician, or cardiologist.

BRAIN TUMOR

Brain tumor is a rare cause of headache, but it is often a major concern of the headache patient. Recent onset of headache or a change in the character of a current headache (especially in those older than age 40) suggests the possibility of a brain tumor. The headache associated with a brain tumor tends to be constant and usually dull in nature rather than severe or knifelike. This headache is made worse by coughing, sneezing, or straining as during a bowel movement, since these all raise the fluid pressure in the brain (also known as cerebral spinal fluid). It may interfere with sleeping and awaken the patient. Pain is typically worse in the morning. If a headache is accompanied by vomiting, blurred vision, lethargy, fainting, dizziness, or personality change, then it becomes mandatory to search for a brain tumor. In most chronic headache patients where a diagnosis is not apparent, CAT scan (Computerized Axial Tomography) of the brain or an MRI (Magnetic Resonance Imaging) study will be requested by the physician in order to visualize the brain and identify a possible lesion or growth.

EYE PROBLEMS

Eye problems are also a rare cause of headache. The discomfort is usually just above the eyes. When headache is related to eye strain, the symptoms are often first noted late in the afternoon (rather than in the morning), after you have been using your eyes all day. Examples of patients who are at increased risk to have headaches secondary to eye strain are college students with long hours of studying, people who sit in front of a computer screen all day, and individuals who drive all day. If you have pressure in or about the eyes, examination by an eye specialist is advised. It is important to check for increased eye or intraocular pressure, which can be seen with glaucoma. More important, there can be errors of refraction (or sight), which may indicate a need for glasses or for a change in your current prescription. There are also some specific inflammations of the eye, for example, optic neuritis, which may result in ocular pain. Remember that some migraine headaches are associated with visual symptoms at their onset. (This will be addressed later in the chapter.)

DENTAL ORIGIN

Head pain with dental origin may be apparent when it occurs in the teeth, especially in the lowers. When biting or chewing causes pain, or any tooth is sensitive to cold food or liquid, you should probably see your dentist. Pain in an upper tooth is usually a dental problem but may also be a sign of disease in an adjacent maxillary (cheek) sinus. The patient with a lingering upper respiratory infection who develops pain in an upper tooth may need sinus rather than dental treatment. Too often I have seen one or more upper teeth extracted in a vain effort to relieve pain that originated in the sinus, or which was a manifestation of trigeminal neuralgia (described later in this chapter).

Somewhat less obvious is the pain that accompanies temporomandibular joint (TMJ) dysfunction. These are the joints where the mandible (jaw) hinges in front of each ear. Abnormal function of these joints may result in ear or jaw pain that is aggravated by chewing or yawning. Additional symptoms include a clicking or popping noise in the involved joints. There may be fullness in the ear or limitation of motion when opening the mouth wide. Patients with TMJ problems often present a history of grinding their teeth, behavior frequently triggered by underlying stress. TMJ disorders commonly occur in people who are missing some back teeth and in those with malocclusion (overbite or underbite).

The use of a night-guard dental splint may be helpful in relieving temporomandibular joint discomfort, especially in anyone who grinds his teeth. Self-help measures include application of heat via a heating pad or hot compresses to the upper jaw to relax adjacent muscles that may be in spasm. A diet of soft food should be implemented and gum chewing should be stopped. If needed, anti-inflammatory medications, such as aspirin or ibuprofen, can be used. Dental rehabilitation may include correction of an abnormal bite or fitting of a partial or full denture to replace missing teeth. Your general dentist or a TMJ specialist can help you with this.

NEURALGIA

This general term refers to pain that occurs when a nerve fires abnormally, producing pain in the area supplied by the nerve. Neuralgia may occur in almost any part of the body. For the purposes of our discussion of headaches, a condition called trigeminal neuralgia will be considered, since this is the primary neuralgia that involves the face and head. This painful disorder is also known as tic douloureux.

The trigeminal—the prefix "tri-" referring to its three divisions—nerve supplies sensation to most of the face. The upper division supplies sensation to the forehead area; the middle division, to that part of the face between the eyes and lips; the third division, from the lips to the chin.

The pain of trigeminal neuralgia is severe, sharp, occurs in paroxysms, and lasts only a few minutes. It may occur in any part of the face depending on which division of the trigeminal nerve is firing abnormally. The most common location is in the middle part of the face, adjacent to the nose or cheek.

These patients usually exhibit a trigger zone, with the pain triggered by irritating a certain spot. Trigger factors may include chewing, shaving, brushing the teeth, or even blowing the nose. Thus, individuals may develop a fear that one of these actions may precipitate a paroxysm of pain. Beginning usually in mid- or late life, the attacks tend to become more severe and more frequent. Examination and X rays are unrevealing, with a diagnosis being made by history alone.

Most trigeminal patients can be managed by prescription medication, but some of the drugs have potent side effects (one drug most commonly used for tic douloureux is an antiseizure medication). As with most recurrent headaches, strong analgesics and narcotics should be avoided, since drug dependency or even addiction is a real possibility. Many of these patients require surgery to destroy the nerve pathway responsible for the neuralgia. This destruction may be by cutting, or by injection with alcohol or boiling water. Additionally, a blood vessel that is pushing on the nerve can be decompressed. Neurosurgical consultation is advised for those patients who continue to have attacks after an adequate trial with medication. However, since neuralgia patients have symptoms of facial pain similar to that caused by sinus or dental infection, it is important for your doctor to be able to differentiate between these, since treatment varies.

MYALGIA

A common type of head pain is myalgia. This muscular discomfort builds gradually, reaches a maximum, and then recedes gradually. It is often brought on by sudden temperature change, especially chills, drafts, or air-conditioning. The muscles affected are often those at the back of the neck. The involved area is tender to touch, with pain often migrating from one area to another. Treatments include application of heat (especially moist heat), use of medication, improved circulation to the affected area, and occasionally muscle relaxants.

ALLERGY

A small number of allergy patients has headache as a primary symptom. You should suspect that allergy is the cause of your headache if it occurs only upon exposure to a certain environment or only after eating a certain food. An example of this allergic headache would be a person who develops headache when exposed to highly scented cosmetics. Cigarette smoke can also be a significant trigger of an allergic headache. When the headache is due to an inhalant, i.e., something breathed in, there is usually nasal congestion and blockage, watery eyes, or other signs of allergy. Food allergies are less obvious. You will have to keep a food diary and note the time of onset of each headache. A pattern may become apparent, with each headache preceded by ingestion of the same offending food. Common food allergens include milk, eggs, wheat, nuts, pork, chocolate, or shellfish.

Avoiding the offending substance is the ideal way to prevent food allergies, but often this is not practical with inhaled substances that may be around you daily or during certain seasons. The use of an antihistamine is helpful. These work by blocking the action of histamine, the substance responsible for allergy symptoms, such as itching, sneezing, watery eyes, and runny nose. Antihistamines that can be purchased without a prescription include Tavist-1, Benadryl, and Chlor-Trimeton. If an antihistamine relieves your headache, suspect allergy as the cause. If an allergic headache is accompanied by nasal congestion, consider an antihistamine-decongestant medication. Examples of this combination include Benadryl Allergy/Sinus caplets, which also contains acetaminophen (Tylenol) for pain relief; Dimetapp, Contact; Tavist-D; and Drixoral Allergy/Sinus. (A more complete list of the medications will be included in Chapter 8.)

OTHER TYPES OF HEADACHES

MIGRAINE

Fred Allen, a famous comedian, once said, "My agent gets 10 percent of everything I get, except my blinding headache." Although the term *migraine* has often been overused, it does correctly refer to one of the more common forms of severe, recurrent headaches. Migraine is categorized as a vascular headache, since it results from distension of blood vessels in the head.

These blood vessels are surrounded by fine nerve fibers, which transmit pain sensations when stretched. Blood coursing through the involved vessel accounts for the throbbing or pulsating quality of a migraine.

The most frequently occurring form of migraine, formerly called common migraine, begins with no aura or warning. The pain is severe, one-sided, and lasts from four to seventy-two hours. It is often accompanied by nausea or vomiting. Movement, bright lights, and loud noise make the headache worse, so these patients seek a quiet, dark place. The headache is usually relieved by sleeping.

The less common form of this disorder is migraine with aura, formerly known as classic migraine. This aura usually takes the form of a visual disturbance, such as blind spots, or shimmering points of light in the field of vision. The aura lasts a matter of minutes, with the headache beginning at the same time or within an hour. Except for the aura, this form of migraine is similar to the more common variety described in the preceding paragraph.

Most migraine patients have an immediate-family member with the same problem, suggesting a genetic factor.

Migraines affect women almost three times as frequently as men. There may be a hormonal influence, since the attacks seem to occur more often during the premenstrual period, and are infrequent after menopause. Fortunately, the headaches are less frequent during pregnancy. Birth control pills should be avoided by the migraine patient. About 20 percent of adults with migraine had their initial attacks before age ten. Another clue to the diagnosis of migraine is that patients may relate a history of motion sickness.

Whereas migraine is an organic headache related to blood-vessel distension, and is different in quality and duration from a tension headache, stress may have a role in the etiology of migraine. This is illustrated by the story of Ulysses S. Grant, the North's leading general during the Civil War. At one point in the later stages of the war, General Grant was suffering a "sick headache" (presumably migraine) for most of the day and night. A messenger arrived with a letter of surrender from Robert E. Lee, chief Confederate general, whereupon General Grant's headache immediately cleared.

Migraine-headache sufferers often will require prescription medication from their physicians. This medication is usually most effective if taken at the onset of the headache rather than later in the course of the attack. Patients with an aura may be able to abort the headache by taking medication at this early warning sign. For years the drugs used to treat migraine often contained ergotamine, an agent that causes blood-vessel constriction (narrowing), thereby counteracting the blood-vessel dilation that is responsible for the pain of this headache. In recent years, the drug Sumatriptan (Imitrex) has been given by injection or orally to abort migraine headache. This medication is more effective than ergotamine and has fewer side effects but is significantly more expensive.

When migraine attacks occur two or more times a week or are not effectively controlled by drugs given at the time of the headache, a course of prophylactic, or preventive, medication may be prescribed. These drugs, for example, Propranolol (Inderal), are taken on a daily basis, often decreasing the frequency and severity of attacks. In some migraine patients, attacks may follow ingestion of certain foods, especially those containing a chemical called tyramine. Foods you should avoid include aged cheese, red wine, chocolate, hot dogs, and certain nuts. MSG, a chemical found in Chinese food, can also bring on a migraine headache. Other nondrug treatments for the person with recurrent migraine may include biofeedback and stress management.

TENSION HEADACHE

The most common cause of chronic, recurrent headaches is the tension headache. While not as severe as the pain of migraine, it tends to be more generalized and characterized by a "tight" or "bandlike" quality. It occurs mainly in adults, often beginning in middle age, and is associated with anxiety and depression. It is infrequent in children and adolescents. Both men and women are affected, the latter somewhat more commonly. Tension headaches can occur on a daily basis for months or years. They may occur across the forehead or temple, over the top of the head, or in the upper neck at the back of the head. The latter is often associated with tightness in the muscles of the neck. Surprisingly, these headaches rarely disturb sleep patterns.

Before the diagnosis of tension headache is made, these patients may require a comprehensive examination, including appropriate X-ray scans or imaging studies, to ensure that there is no underlying, organic basis for the headache. In many patients, sources of psychologic stress are uncovered: marital problems or job stress. Many of these patients suffer depression and anxiety. In the past, tension headaches were attributed to excessive muscle contraction or restriction of scalp arteries, but this theory is no longer in vogue. Certainly, anyone with recurrent headaches from any cause may exhibit some muscle tension.

Most tension headache patients have a long history of taking over-the-counter analgesics. Treatment begins when the patient, after a complete examination, is reassured that there is no serious underlying physical cause for the headaches. Relaxation is the key to long-term relief, but some type of anxiety-relieving medication must usually be prescribed. Strong pain medication, especially narcotics or other addictive drugs, must be avoided. Alternative, non-medication treatments that may be helpful in reducing tension headaches include massage, heat, and biofeedback. Acupuncture has been used with some success but must be administered by someone well trained and having extensive experience in this ancient art.

CLUSTER HEADACHE

Next in frequency of occurrence after migraine and tension headaches are cluster types. These are intense in character and one-sided in location. Cluster headache is steady rather than throbbing, as with migraine, and is often accompanied by tearing and watery nasal discharge, with congestion on the same side as the headache. Whereas migraine is usually a female disorder, more than 80 percent of cluster headache patients are male. Another significant feature is that this headache usually occurs at night, often waking the victim one to two hours into sleep. The episodes occur for several weeks to months, lasting up to one hour. They tend to occur in the same pattern many months or years later.

While the exact cause of cluster headache is unknown, it is associated with dilated blood vessels. Unlike migraine, there is rarely an element of tension involved, nor is there a family history of similar headaches. Alcoholic beverages, with their tendency to dilate blood vessels, should be avoided by anyone with cluster headaches. Prescribed medication, including narcotics, may be needed to provide relief for those with cluster headaches.

GENERAL APPROACH TO
AND TREATMENT OF HEADACHES

We have discusssed many types of headaches, although a complete review of the topic could easily fill several volumes. The various disorders previously outlined are noted to help the sinus headache patient better define and get at the true cause of his head pain. Often, what a patient believes is a sinus headache turns out to have a different etiology. The importance of describing for your physician the location, character, duration, and frequency of your headache and associated symptoms cannot be overemphasized.

Do not continue to take frequent painkilling medication for headaches without first finding out the cause of the problem. Headache patients may need to visit a neurologist (brain and nervous-system specialist), otorhinolaryngologist (ear, nose, and throat specialist), ophthalmologist (eye specialist), dentist, or possibly a psychiatrist to help with their problems. A plan of action should be devised to prevent or at least minimize the attacks. If a thorough search for organic disease has ruled out the presence of a physical cause, be willing to accept the diagnosis of tension or psychogenic headache.

Table 6.1 lists commonly advertised, nonprescription products for headache relief. Note that every product listed contains either aspirin or acetaminophen, an aspirin substitute; some contain both.

Aspirin is truly a wonder drug and a fine analgesic. Some recent studies have shown that it is as effective for pain relief as the most popular prescription pain pill. The only drugs that are stronger than aspirin are those containing codeine or other addictive narcotics. Aspirin tablets, regardless of brand, are identical in strength (300 milligrams) and effectiveness. Price is the major variant and relates more to the cost of advertising a product than to its contents.

How about buffered aspirin? Several products in Table 6.1 contain aspirin, plus an antacid. Since aspirin is an acid substance, it will cause stomach upset in some individuals. These people should probably use a buffered product, as should those who may be taking six or more aspirins daily, for instance, patients with arthritis. While buffered aspirin is more rapidly absorbed into the bloodstream than regular aspirin, the onset of analgesic action is not of any clinical significance. If you are taking buffered aspirin to decrease gastric upset, then its higher cost is

Table 6.1   Nonprescription Headache Products

BRAND NAME	ANALGESIC CONTENT	OTHER INGREDIENTS
Alka-Seltzer	Aspirin	Antacid, citric acid
Anacin	Aspirin	Caffeine
Ascriptin	Aspirin	Antacids
BC	Aspirin, salicylamide	Caffeine
Bromo-Seltzer	Acetaminophen	Antacids, sodium citrate
Bufferin	Aspirin	Antacids
Empirin	Aspirin, phenacetin	Caffeine
Excedrin	Acetaminophen, aspirin, salicylamide	Caffeine
Vanquish	Acetaminophen	Sodium citrate

worthwhile; if you are taking the buffered product for its faster action, don't bother.

Many patients cannot take aspirin due to gastric distress: They have a history of stomach ulcers, allergy to aspirin, or because they are on a blood thinner (the aspirin causes additional blood thinning and can be problematic in these patients). Acetaminophen is an aspirin substitute, to be taken in the same dosage of two tablets every four hours as needed. Common brands of acetaminophen are Tylenol, Datril, Tempro, or Valadol.

Notice how many of the listed headache products contain additional ingredients. This adds to the cost and increases the likelihood of side effects. Pharmaceutical companies continue to juggle these ingredients to give the illusion that their formula offers new hope for the headache sufferer. Stick with aspirin—buffered aspirin if needed—or acetaminophen.

The deception of the public is best illustrated by one of the most famous names in Table 6.1 (my lawyer advises that it remains anonymous). The original formula of this "wonder" pain pill contained aspirin, caffeine, and acetanilid, a drug that could produce serious blood problems with prolonged use. Eventually, acetanilid was removed, and an analgesic called phenacetin was inserted. Many millions of tablets later, it was learned that phenacetin could cause kidney failure, so it was removed. Now this widely advertised product contains aspirin and caffeine, the later equivalent to one-fourth cup of coffee. Although the aspirin content of the product is only about 20 percent more than in a regular aspirin tablet, its cost is four times as much as generic aspirin. Throughout these multiple changes in content, the well-advertised brand name remained the same. Only the most careful label reader might have been aware of the changes.

For most headaches, aspirin will suffice. If two tablets do not provide three to four hours of relief of your headache, seek medical advice.

CONCLUSION

This chapter has explored the frequent types of headaches, so that the sinus headache patient may better define and understand the true cause of his pain. As mentioned, it is important for you to carefully describe your headache to your physician so that he can help diagnose and treat you appropriately. While headache patients are a major segment of the sinus population, so too are children. The next chapter will examine pediatric sinus disease, with emphasis on related conditions and treatment.

SINUS DISEASE IN CHILDREN

While a runny nose in a child is typically a sign of a common cold, persistent congestion may indicate a sinus infection. Even though the sinuses are not fully developed in children, recognition of sinus infection is important so that a search for contributing factors can be undertaken and appropriate treatment be given. This chapter will examine these factors specific to children and suggest proper treatment for childhood sinusitis.

SINUS DEVELOPMENT IN CHILDREN

At birth, only the ethmoid (the sinuses between the eyes) and maxillary (cheek) sinuses are present, and at that time they're the size of a pea. The sphenoid sinus (behind the eyes) begins to grow at age two and is not even apparent on X rays until age five. The frontal (forehead) sinus is the last to develop, at about age four. Most of these paranasal sinuses reach adult size by adolescence, with the frontals growing until age twenty.

For this reason, the sinuses most commonly involved in infections are the maxillary and ethmoid, with the frontal and sphenoid becoming involved in late childhood and adolescence. Immaturity of the sinus cavities in infants makes sinus X rays of little use at this age.

THE RUNNY-NOSE CHILD

We are all familiar with the child like Jordan, a three-year-old patient who, all winter long, sniffles and rubs his nose on his shirtsleeve. His parents seem to be forever wiping mucus as it drips from his nose, and encouraging him to try to blow.

Several things can cause a constant runny nose in children. Normally, children have six to eight upper respiratory infections (i.e., colds) each year. Only a small percentage of these colds leads to an actual sinus infection. However, these colds account for an estimated twenty-six million missed school days. Children in day-care settings seem to be at an increased risk of upper respiratory infections, but with many mothers working today, day care is often a necessity and a difficult situation to alter.

Aside from the common cold, allergies are probably the next greatest cause of the runny-nosed child. Allergies may occur during certain seasons of the year (termed *seasonal allergies*) or throughout the year (termed *perennial allergies*). Allergy causes swelling of the nasal and sinus linings, and results in a watery nasal discharge or drip. This allergic congestion is one factor that may lead to sinus infection.

Sinus infection is another cause of childhood runny nose and should be considered if the nasal drainage lasts longer than the seven to ten-day uncomplicated viral cold. However, the criteria for sinusitis in children is more stringent than in adults, primarily because upper respiratory illness so frequently occurs in the normal child. Sinusitis in children is not even termed chronic until symptoms persist for three months or longer (in adults, sinusitis is termed chronic after six weeks).

A number of conditions in children, rarely seen in adults, can lead to excessive nasal drainage. One of these is adenoiditis, meaning "inflammation of the adenoids." The adenoids sit in the back of the nose in an area called the nasopharynx (refer to Figure 4.3 on page 57). In children, they can be large and manifested by loud snoring and a nasal voice. Adenoids tend to shrink during the teenage years, and are usually gone by age eighteen. Chronic infection of the adenoids can itself cause a runny nose, or may secondarily infect the sinuses. Large tonsils or chronic tonsil infection can also lead to sinus infections in children. A rare congenital condition, usually diagnosed early in life, is called *choanal atresia,* in which there is blockage at the back of the nasal passages. If there is a narrowing rather than complete blockage, we use the term *choanal stenosis.* When this occurs, the mucus that the nose and sinuses produce cannot drain backward and thus pours out the front of the nose.

Every so often I see a child like Laura, a two-year-old who, for several weeks, had foul-smelling drainage from one side of her nose. After two courses of antibiotics had no effect, her pediatrician referred her to me. Other than her older brother, who recently had suffered through the flu, her parents could not figure out what was causing her problems. When I got a close look inside her nose in my office, I pulled from her left nostril a small button, surrounded by a thick, yellow crust. Her problems soon went away. When young children or the mentally retarded have one-sided nasal drainage, consider that it could be a foreign body in the nose. Other examples of commonly found nasal foreign bodies include peanuts, raisins, popcorn, crayon pieces, and beads.

CHILDHOOD ALLERGY

Although Chapter 6 of this book deals entirely with allergy, some specific points pertain to the pediatric population. While it is important to differentiate allergy from "sinus disease," you must realize that in some individuals, the two are closely linked, with allergy being the primary cause of sinus ostia swelling, blockage, and infection. Thus, the allergy component must be treated to improve the sinus condition.

Aside from the typical allergy symptoms of thin, watery drainage, sneezing, and watery eyes, the allergic child may manifest some other common traits. Children often give the "allergic salute"—upward rubbing of their draining nose. Dark circles around the eyes, termed *allergic shiners* (or "black eyes of allergy") may be present. Allergic children may also have ear symptoms of chronic infection, or lung problems with cough and asthma. Eczema also indicates that allergies are playing a role in the child's symptoms.

Another clue to allergy in children is family history. If

both parents have a history of allergy, there is a 65 to 75 percent chance that the child will have allergies. An allergic sibling also should raise your index of suspicion. The family history may also include allergy-related diseases like asthma or eczema.

Allergy-testing is difficult in children, but it can be done by either skin-testing or by a blood test (RAST). (These tests are more fully described in Chapter 6.) Whereas allergy-testing may be necessary in patients whose symptoms cannot be controlled with medication, many allergic children can be managed by a combination of nasal allergy sprays and oral antihistamines. Antihistamines, with and without decongestants, traditionally cause drowsiness in adults, yet, paradoxically in some children, cause hyperactivity. Cortisone-containing (steroid) nasal sprays are generally not recommended for use in children younger than six.

DIAGNOSIS OF CHILDHOOD SINUS DISEASE

Diagnosing sinus disease in children is more difficult than in adults. First of all, children are tougher to examine. Symptoms of childhood sinusitis can be more subtle than in adults. In addition, children are often unable to describe what they are feeling. However, if you notice a number of the following features in your child, it may indicate a sinus condition:

- Anytime an upper respiratory infection lasts more than ten to fourteen days, it is likely developing into a sinus infection.

- If your child's nose is constantly running, especially

thick, yellow or green mucus, he may have a chronic sinus condition. The nasal drainage may also be post-nasal and drip into the throat.

* While a child may not report this postnasal drip, he may likely have a chronic cough of unclear origin. This cough often occurs at night, when the child is lying down, and can disrupt sleep. It can also occur first thing in the morning, when the child awakens.

* This postnasal drainage may further lead to bad breath (in medical terms, called *halitosis*).

* Postnasal drip can also lead to sore throat.

* When the child swallows this constant mucous stream, he can have nausea and vomit.

* Headaches, a common complaint of the adult sinus patient, are rarely expressed before age six.

* While adults report feeling "run-down" from pro-longed sinus infection, children may instead show behavioral changes, irritability, and fatigue.

* Complications of sinus infection include spreading to the nearby eye structures, with resultant eye swelling and drainage, or spreading to the brain and sur-rounding structures. Although these complications (especially the orbital problems) occur more fre-quently in children than in adults, they are still rare, especially today when antibiotics are given early in the course of the illness.

Clues to Sinus Infection in Children

- thick nasal drainage (from the front of the nose)
- postnasal drip (down the throat)
- cough
- bad breath
- sore throat
- headache or head pain
- nausea/vomiting
- behavioral changes
- high fever (rare)
- orbital swelling/complications (rare)

CHILDREN AT RISK FOR SINUSITIS

There are several specific groups of children who are at increased risk of sinus disease:

- As mentioned earlier in this chapter, allergies are inter-related to sinus disease. Allergic children comprise a large number of the pediatric sinus population.

- Children with chronic adenoid and tonsil infections may also have chronic sinusitis. Stagnated tonsil and adenoid infection can act as a primary source for chronic sinus infection, or may secondarily block the sinus openings, with resultant infection. Studies have been done where children appeared to have a sinus infection, with clouding of the sinuses on X ray. Once the tonsils and adenoids were removed, the children's symptoms disappeared, and their X rays completely normalized.

105

- Cleft palate or other facial defects can lead to alterations in sinus development and drainage, and lead to infection.

- There are a number of defects in mucous clearance with abnormal hair cells (the hair cells normally move mucus through the nose and sinuses). These often present themselves early in life as childhood diseases. For example, in a disease called ciliary dyskinesia (meaning abnormal hair-cell movement), there is poor mucus drainage, with more resultant sinus infections. Although most of these conditions are rare, it is important to keep them in mind, especially if your child seems to have constant sinus infections, and responds poorly to standard medical treatment.

- Cystic fibrosis, a hereditary illness of abnormal gland function, is found primarily in the pediatric population. These children, who typically die by their twenties, are plagued by digestive and lung problems, and additionally by chronic sinusitis and nasal polyps. Cystic fibrosis patients have abnormally thickened mucus, leading to blockage of the sinus ostia, and infection.

- Children with underlying lung problems seem at risk for sinus disease. The most frequent illness of this category is asthma. The lung linings and the lining of the nose are abnormal in the asthmatic child, and the sinuses are hyperreactive. Additionally, a sinus infection with postnasal drainage can exacerbate childhood asthma.

- Many diseases, often hereditary, involve immature or inadequate immune systems. Children with these problems may be missing one or more types of cells that ward off offending agents. This class of diseases, for example, immunoglobulin deficiencies, should be considered if your child seems to get a variety of different types of infections. A series of blood tests can identify the problem.

- Another factor that can contribute to sinus disease and is often forgotten (or overlooked) in children is secondhand smoke. A household filled with smoke may lead to swelling and irritation of the nasal lining, as well as altered cilia (hair) function, with resultant sinus blockage and infection. Similarly, children who have a parent who smokes (and thus are exposed to secondhand smoke) are at risk for pediatric ear infections.

- In recent years, the importance of gastroesophageal reflux (termed GER) in upper airway disease has been recognized. GER, most often seen in infants, occurs when stomach acid backs up into the esophagus (food pipe). This reflux can trigger symptoms as far up as the throat or even the nasopharynx. Often, a child will not have symptoms of reflux like heartburn or vomiting, but may instead have hoarseness, cough, or irregular breathing. Physicians have reported cases of children with chronic nasal and sinus symptoms, which decreased dramatically after their reflux was treated.

TREATMENT OF
CHILDHOOD SINUS DISEASE

If you suspect that your child has a chronic or recurring sinus condition based on the symptoms described above, there are a number of things you can do on your own that might lessen the problem.

If allergy seems to be a strong component, try to identify allergic triggers. Food allergies can be avoided. Environmental factors like dust or mold can be minimized (see Chapter 5). If your child seems to have sinus infections since you brought home a new dog or cat three months ago, you may have to think about getting rid of your pet.

Sometimes sinus problems worsen in the winter months, when dry air leads to poor mucous clearance in the nose and sinuses. A humidifier or vaporizer placed in a child's room at night can increase the moisture in the air (this is more fully explained in Chapter 2). Moisture can be added either as cool air with a humidifier, or as warm steam with a vaporizer. Many people find the hot steam more soothing. However, with young children, a cool-mist humidifier may be preferable, since the child may sustain burns from tipping over a steam vaporizer.

As described earlier in this chapter, secondhand smoke can make sinus disease worse. If you cannot quit smoking, at least make it a policy for all smokers to go outside of the house, away from children when smoking. And please, no smoking in the closed quarters of a car. Also, make sure there are no smokers at day-care or baby-sitting facilities. Don't forget that smoking has become a popular habit among teenagers and can be a contributing factor in your teen's sinusitis.

You may suspect that gastroesophageal reflux is playing a factor in your child's health problems, especially if he is frequently vomiting or spitting up. Reflux is more common in young infants and often resolves as the child gets older. Initial treatment of GER in children can begin with simple measures, like elevating the head of the bed, eliminating bedtime feedings, and thickening your child's feedings with products such as cereal. Persistent symptoms warrant a physician's evaluation, which may include X-ray studies (such as a barium swallow or a nuclear milk scan). Medications may be needed, and typically control symptoms. Surgery is reserved for rare situations, when reflux is severe and unresponsive to conservative measures.

OVER-THE-COUNTER MEDICATIONS FOR CHILDHOOD SINUSITIS

Although your child may not tell you if he feels uncomfortable with the nasal congestion or sore throat that accompanies his sinus infection, most parents have a sense of when their child is struggling. If their simple cold is causing crankiness or persistent symptoms, you may want to start an over-the-counter medication to prevent what may turn into—or may already have turned into—a sinus infection.

Decongestants
Decongestants act to decrease swelling in the nose and aid in airflow, as well as sinus drainage. Decongestants come in two forms—oral (pills) and topical (drops or sprays). Oral decongestants may work well in the nose but can also have the central (brain) effect of causing hyperactivity in some children; this factor often may limit their use in some

children. For this reason, topical decongestant nose drops may prove more useful in some cases. However, there are several cautions about nasal drops in children: The drops or sprays are not typically recommended for children younger than five, and may be difficult to instill in the fighting child. They should only be used in certain situations, and not for more than five days, since they can cause a rebound swelling in the nose. Despite these limitations, decongestant drops or sprays are helpful when the child is extremely uncomfortable because he cannot breathe out of his nose; they can relieve the congestion and allow the child to get some sleep.

Antihistamines

Antihistamines counteract allergy symptoms. Although they can decrease the possible allergy component in pediatric sinus disease, antihistamines can dry up the mucus so much that the child is left with thickened mucus that will not drain out of the nose and sinuses. While most over-the-counter antihistamines cause drowsiness in adults, they may have the paradoxical effect of agitation in children. As happens with decongestants, this may prove the medications intolerable (especially to the parents of the wound-up child).

Analgesics

General discomfort can be decreased with an analgesic product. Aspirin should be avoided in children, since it can cause a rare but serious complication called Reye's syndrome. Instead, products containing acetaminophen (for example, Children's Tylenol) or ibuprofen (for example, Children's Advil) should be used.

Cough Medications

The last major category of over-the-counter sinus medication for children are the cough medications. Most useful are those agents containing guaifenesin, a compound termed a *mucolytic,* which act to thin mucus and help the child expectorate or cough it up.

Combination Products

Many of these over-the-counter (OTC) medications come as combinations. Try only to use those products that contain what the child really needs, since additional compounds have additional side effects. (A complete listing of OTC medications is included in Chapter 8.) Pediatric doses are typically based on weight. If you are unable to figure out from the package insert (often based on standard average weight for specific ages) the dose to give your child, check with your pharmacist or contact your doctor.

SEEING THE DOCTOR

At what point in your child's upper respiratory infection should you see the doctor for a possible sinus infection? If cold symptoms persist more than a week, or if your child seems to be developing a complication such as an earache, sore throat, or high fever, it is probably wise to make a visit to your pediatrician or family practitioner. For the acute infection, a one- to two-week course of an antibiotic will likely be prescribed. Additional prescription medications, such as decongestants, antihistamines, and cough suppressants, may be recommended based on your child's symptoms. An X ray or culture is typically unnecessary for the uncomplicated acute sinusitis in a child.

Chronic sinus symptoms can be subtle in a child, so it is sometimes difficult for a parent to know when to seek medical evaluation. Once symptoms such as cough or rhinorrhea (runny nose) persist for several weeks and seem to be causing discomfort, seek your doctor's advice. Initial treatment of chronic sinusitis in children should involve rigorous medical therapy. This includes a long-term course of antibiotics. The antibiotic should cover a wide range of sinus organisms and be used for three to six weeks, or longer. Nasal steroid sprays can be used safely for children older than six to shrink the lining of the nose and sinuses and aid in sinus drainage. As in acute sinus infections, your child's doctor may prescribe additional medications (for example, decongestants, antihistamines, mucous-thinning agents, or combination products) to help with symptoms. Often this longer course of medication will clear up the child's chronic sinus disease. If you have trouble getting your child to take medication, let the doctor know so that he can prescribe once-daily medications if possible.

If, despite adequate medical therapy, symptoms persist, it is time to look closely for underlying causes for the sinusitis. As mentioned earlier in this chapter, these may include allergies, secondhand smoke (or firsthand smoke in teenagers), gastroesophageal reflux, or an underlying medical condition or anatomic abnormality.

At this point in your child's illness, the doctor may order an X-ray study. Plain sinus X rays may show sinus disease but are of little help in the child where all the sinuses are not fully developed. Rather, a CT (also known as a CAT scan) X ray of the sinuses is of greater use in evaluating structural problems. Currently, with newer high-tech scanners, these can be carried out relatively quickly in children, with sedation usually needed only in infants to keep them still. These newer generations of scanners also have even less radiation than plain sinus X rays and yield much more information, especially in children where the paranasal sinus development is not fully complete. If an underlying anatomical problem is found and the child has failed maximal medical therapy, then he may be a candidate for surgical treatment.

SURGERY FOR PEDIATRIC SINUSITIS

As a mother myself, I can understand most parents' fear of having their child undergo an operation. However, there are a number of instances when surgery should be considered. If a child is having a complication of sinusitis, such as orbital abscess or severe brain infection, then sinus drainage may be indicated. Another indication for surgical treatment of sinus disease is "medical therapy failures." In other words, if your child has been on many months of many different medications without relief, it may be time to think about surgery. Sinus procedures should be performed in cases in which quality of life is altered by the sinus disease. Quality of life may be more difficult to define in the child than in the adult but may be assumed in cases of severe nasal obstruction or drainage, persistent pain, or generalized illness. If your child has underlying lung disease that is worsened by constant sinus infection and postnasal drip, then his doctor may recommend a surgical procedure. Examples are patients with asthma or cystic fibrosis. Studies of asthmatic children with sinusitis have found fewer emergency room visits and a sharp decrease in inhalers after their sinuses were treated surgically. However, surgery should be considered as a last resort.

Criteria for Surgery for Pediatric Sinusitis

- complications
- failure of medical therapy
- if sinus disease aggravates lung disease (examples: asthma, cystic fibrosis)
- quality of life

Once you and your child's doctor decide that surgery is warranted, what type of operation should be done? A number of different procedures may be offered, some aimed directly at the sinuses themselves and others that indirectly help sinusitis by improving drainage. While Chapter 10 fully describes sinus surgery in the adult, we will now concentrate on surgery for the child. Many factors are specific to the treatment of children. Whereas adult sinus surgery can often be performed under general (full) anesthesia or local anesthesia with sedation (medications are given through an IV in the arm to make you groggy), children almost always require a general anesthetic. Some doctors even feel that some of these procedures (for example, endoscopic surgery—covered later in this chapter) may require a second anesthetic for postoperative care of the nasal and sinus cavities. Additionally, the paranasal sinuses may not yet be fully developed in the pediatric surgery patient, making some of the procedures that are useful in adults less helpful in the child. Since allergy often has an important role in childhood sinusitis, allergies must also be treated adequately to allow for optimal results following surgery.

Adenoidectomy and Tonsillectomy

As discussed, adenoids, which sit in the back of the nose in the nasopharynx, can be a major contributor to sinus disease in children. A key to large adenoids may be loud snoring and mouth breathing. This may be verified by an X ray called the lateral neck film or examination by your doctor. However, it is not the size of the adenoids alone that is important. Sometimes, the adenoids may not be large but may harbor chronic infection through blockage of the sinus openings in the nose.

Surgery to remove the adenoids is called adenoidectomy. It is a relatively safe operation in children older than two but may be performed on younger children if needed. The adenoids are typically removed through the mouth by mirror visualization. They are usually scraped out with instruments, and the area is cauterized for bleeding. Less commonly, they are taken out with a laser through the nose, although this can sometimes lead to complications like scarring. Adenoidectomy is rarely accompanied by postoperative bleeding and has a short recovery period, with little discomfort.

The role that the tonsils (located in the back of the mouth) play in sinusitis is still unclear. If they are large and recurrently infected, then the tonsils are likely contributing to sinus infection. Removal of the tonsils, although typically performed on an outpatient basis, is more involved than adenoidectomy, with sore throat lasting up to a week.

Correction of a Deviated Septum

The nasal septum, which is the cartilage and bony wall separating the two sides of the nose, can be deviated (or twisted), leading to sinusitis by blocking the sinus ostia (drainage areas). Correction of this problem is called septoplasty or submucous resection, an outpatient procedure requiring packing in the nose for at least one day. Since surgery on the septum may affect facial growth, it is rarely advised in children before age sixteen (roughly following the child's growth spurt). In those infrequent situations in which marked deviation of the septum causes nasal or sinus disease in children, surgery is performed in a conservative fashion, removing as little cartilage and bone as possible.

"Draining the Sinuses"

In certain situations, a procedure called antral lavage is performed. This involves lavaging or "washing out" the antrum, which is another name for the maxillary or cheek sinus. A needle is placed through the nose into the maxillary sinus to wash it out of infections. This does not provide long-term benefit but may clear out a collection of pus that is not responding to antibiotics. Sinus lavage does provide a way to obtain material from the sinus for culture in the very sick patient (often a patient with a deficient immune system). Sometimes your doctor may recommend antral lavage to clean out the sinuses at the same time that a child is under anesthesia for adenoidectomy.

Nasal Antral Window

Another procedure utilized in children with sinus disease that is unresponsive to medications is called a "nasal antral window." This is performed through the nose, where an opening is made between the nose and the antrum (the maxillary sinus). This results in permanent ventilation of the sinus through this "window" between the nose and the maxillary sinus (refer to Figure 1.3 on page 5). This window prevents filling of the sinus with mucus and pus during subsequent upper respiratory infections.

While this procedure is relatively easy to perform through the nose, it typically must be done under general anesthesia. These windows have a tendency to close, and may not offer a permanent solution to chronic sinus problems. There is also the potential for injury to developing teeth, since upper tooth roots may lie in the floor of the maxillary sinus.

Caldwell-Luc Operation

Sinus problems in children may warrant procedures directed at specific sinuses. An example of this is the Caldwell-Luc procedure, where an incision is made under the gum to get into the maxillary sinus. This is utilized in situations of chronic maxillary sinus infection, allowing for direct visualization of the sinus. However, because the sinus may not yet be fully developed in the child, there is the possible risk of interrupting normal sinus growth or normal dentition (secondary teeth that are developing are at risk).

External Ethmoid Sinus Drainage

External surgery to drain the ethmoid sinuses (sinuses between the eyes) is termed an *external ethmoidectomy.* Currently, ethmoid sinus disease can be approached through the nose, and so this external surgery, which leaves a scar on the face, is usually used only in those cases where there has been a serious orbital (eye) complication of sinus disease.

Endoscopic Sinus Surgery

In the past decade, the philosophy of sinus surgery has shifted from external surgeries on diseased sinuses to "functional" procedures, aimed at restoring normal sinus function and drainage. These procedures are termed *functional endoscopic sinus surgery*, as they are performed with an endoscope or telescope through the nose. There are fewer complications in these intranasal procedures when performed by an experienced sinus surgeon. Recuperation is typically easier than with external procedures. Endoscopic surgery involves removing diseased tissue of the ethmoid sinus and creating an opening (called a window or antrostomy) between the maxillary sinus and its natural drainage opening into the nose beneath the middle turbinate bone (see Figure 1.3 on page 5).

The philosophy and technique of endoscopic sinus surgery, which is currently the standard procedure in the United States, is described in detail in Chapter 10. There are a few variations to remember in children. First, intranasal surgery in children whose nasal passages and paranasal sinuses are still developing can be difficult and should not be taken lightly. Additionally, postoperative cleaning and suctioning of the sinus cavities is important, especially to prevent the formation of scar bands. While it can be performed in the office setting in teenagers and adults, this post-op cleaning may require a second anesthetic agent in a child, who will typically not sit still for a telescopic exam in the office. Therefore, you should feel comfortable that you have exhausted all other options (including medications and allergy treatment) before allowing your child to undergo surgery on his sinuses.

Sinus Surgery in Children

- adenoidectomy +/− tonsillectomy

- septoplasty (to correct deviated septum)

- antral lavage (sinus "wash")

- nasal antral window

- Caldwell-Luc

- external ethmoidectomy

- endoscopic sinus surgery
  (endoscopic ethmoidectomy and middle meatus nasal antral window)

CONCLUSION

Sinus disease in children, while in some ways similar to that in adults, has a number of factors specific to the pediatric population. Symptoms can be subtle, making diagnosis difficult. The role of allergy and frequent upper respiratory infections in children should be considered. Surgical options should be used only if long-term medical therapy fails to provide relief.

MEDICATIONS FOR THE NOSE AND SINUSES

T here are probably more nonprescription medications for the nose and sinuses than any other part of the body. In 1994 more than four billion dollars was spent on cold, sinus, allergy, and cough products. However, all this money is not necessarily well-spent. In a poll of pharmacists regarding which product categories cause confusion among consumers, allergy relief, cough, and cold preparations top the list, with sinus remedies close behind.

In a survey on self-medication comparing fourteen countries, the United States led the list in percent of consumers using nonprescription medication. Lower cost is the reason most often given for using these products, followed by convenience and eliminating the need for a doctor's visit. If you are familiar with these products, you will be able to select appropriate ones for relief of your nasal and sinus symptoms. You also need to be aware of potential misuse and side effects of the readily available medications.

The term over-the-counter, designated as OTC, will be used synonymously with nonprescription. In recent years, many drugs that formerly required a prescription have been changed to OTC status. This makes it even more important for you to understand the benefits and limitations of these medicines. Since many sinus problems, especially infection, require prescription drugs, we'll present an overview of categories of medications that your doctor may prescribe. The lists of medications in this chapter are not all-inclusive but are offered to provide a general sense of some of the more popular medicines available in the United States. Their order is purely alphabetical.

NASAL DECONGESTANTS

More than three thousand years ago the Chinese inhaled vapors from a plant called horsetail to relieve congestion. Today we know that this plant contains the drug ephedrine, a decongestant which has the ability to shrink the lining of the nose and facilitate easier breathing. Nasal congestion, with swelling of the lining of the nose, is common to upper respiratory infections such as colds, nasal allergies, and sinusitis. This swelling is largely due to dilated blood vessels within the nasal lining. Nasal decongestants shrink the swollen lining by stimulating receptors in the blood-vessel wall to contract. Decongestants come in oral and topical forms (sprays, drops) that work directly on the nasal lining.

ORAL DECONGESTANTS

The two most common oral forms of decongestants are pseudoephedrine and phenylpropanolamine. The latter, in addition to its decongestant properties, is also used as an appetite suppressant. Both drugs are found in many non-prescription product combinations. The most readily available decongestant, with no additional ingredients, is Sudafed™, a trade name of psuedoephedrine. This can be purchased in 30 or 60 mg tablets, or in a 30 mg per teaspoon liquid form for children. Table 8.1 outlines dosages that can be given every four to six hours.

TABLE 8.1   Recommended Dosages for Oral Decongestants

AGE	TSP. OF SYRUP	30 MG TABLETS	60 MG TABLETS
2 to 5 years	—	—	—
6 to 12 years	1	1	—
12 years or older	2	2	1

Sudafed twelve-hour caplets are available for adult use only. The primary side effects of pseudoephedrine and other decongestant-containing tablets is an increase in heart rate and blood pressure, and stimulation of the central nervous system. This stimulation may take the form of nervousness, dizziness, or sleeplessness. These drugs should

be avoided by patients with high blood pressure, heart disease, diabetes, or thyroid disorders, since they can worsen
these conditions. They should also be avoided by patients
taking any of the group of drugs known as monoamine
oxidase inhibitors. In people who are kept awake by
decongestants, take the last dose by six P.M. Since decongestants have an adverse effect on men with prostate
enlargement, they should be taken in smaller doses in
men older than sixty, and the sustained twelve-hour form
should be avoided.

TOPICAL DECONGESTANTS

For those who cannot take oral decongestants for any of the
above reasons, topical decongestants in the form of nose
sprays or nose drops can provide relief. Sprays are somewhat easier to use and offer a better spread of medication
across the lining of the nose. Drops may be easier to use in
infants and young children, since they can be dripped into
the nose. Topical decongestants tend to have fewer side
effects than their oral counterparts, but there is some
absorption of sprays and drops. This is especially true in
infants and children, where there may be excessive absorption of the drug. The side effect of blood-pressure elevation
and rapid pulse can occur with their use, so the same cautions as listed for decongestant tablets apply.

The major caution regarding use of nose sprays or
drops is that use longer than three to five days may result
in rebound. As the effect of a given dose wears off, the
nasal lining swells again. The patient finds that the subsequent doses provide less relief, and a vicious cycle is set
up. This is typified by my patient Gwen, who had been

Table 8.2   Nasal Decongestant Sprays

GENERIC NAME	TRADE NAME	FORMS
Phenylephrine	Neo-Synephrine	*Drops:* 0.125% for infants 0.25% for children 0.5- 1% for adults *Spray:* 0.25% for children 0.5% for adults
	Nostril	*Pump spray:* 0.25% for children 0.5% for adults
	Vicks Sinex	*Spray:* 0.5% for adults
Oxymetazoline *(All oxymetazoline* *preparations should* *be restricted to* *children over 12* *and adults)*	Afrin	*Drops:* 0.05% *Spray:* 0.05% *Nasal Pump Spray:* 0.05%
	Duration	*Spray:* 0.05%
	4-Way Long- lasting Spray	*Spray:* 0.05%
	NTZ	*Spray:* 0.05%
	Neo-Synephrine Maximum Strength	*Spray:* 0.05% *Pump Spray:* 0.05%
	Nostrilla	*Pump Spray:* 0.05%

continued on next page

TABLE 8.2   *continued*

GENERIC NAME	TRADE NAME	FORMS
Oxymetazoline *continued*	Vicks Sinex 12 hour	*Pump Spray:* 0.05%
Xylometazoline	Otrivin	*Drops:* 0.05% for children over 2 0.1% for adults (*Adult preparations can be used by children 12 and over.*) *Spray:* 0.1% for adults

using a nasal decongestant spray every few hours for the past five years yet still felt unable to breathe through her nose. The lining was swollen and inflamed from chronic nose-spray use. I made her throw out her spray while in my office, and had her begin using saline (pure saltwater) sprays. When I saw her a month later, she was feeling great and off all nasal medications.

A minor annoyance of these topical medications may be burning, stinging, or sneezing. These can be minimized by spraying the nose with a saltwater (saline) solution before applying the decongestant. The decongestant drops and sprays listed in Table 8.2 are available without a prescription (list is not all-inclusive). Phenylephrine can be used every four hours if needed. The other products listed have up to twelve hours of action, and should be used twice a day (but only for three to five days). They are intended only for use by children older than twelve and adults.

COLD PREPARATIONS

Most pharmacies have a number of shelves devoted to nonprescription cold or sinus remedies. Almost all of these products have multiple ingredients. They usually contain a decongestant, which helps open clogged nasal passages. Many "cold" tablets or liquids contain an antihistamine. Despite numerous advertisements to the contrary, antihistamines have no legitimate purpose in treating viral illness such as colds or flu. They may decrease a runny nose, since antihistamines have a drying effect. However, this drying of the nasal secretions thickens mucus in the nose and throat, which may result in plugging of the sinuses or blocking of the eustachian tubes. The body's normal defense mechanisms work better when mucus becomes thinner and less viscous. This is best accomplished by increasing your fluid intake, by taking an expectorant such as guaifensein (Robitussin), and by using a humidifier or vaporizer. Another disadvantage of antihistamines is their common side effect of drowsiness. This drowsiness, added to the normal fatigue that comes from an upper respiratory illness, makes it more difficult to maintain your normal activity level. This is especially true for those who drive or who work around machinery. Many cold medications are labeled non-drowsy formula, indicating that they do not contain an antihistamine.

Analgesics, such as aspirin and acetaminophen (Tylenol), may be helpful in lowering fever or in relieving the aches and pains of a viral illness, but they have no direct effect on the viral illness itself. If you do not require medication to lower fever or relieve pain, then don't choose a multi-ingredient product that includes aspirin or acetaminophen with each dosage. For many people, aspirin causes irritation of the stomach lining; in some, bleeding. This side effect can be minimized by taking buffered aspirin (for example, Ascriptin, Bufferin, Bayer Plus), which includes an antacid. Another way to avoid the stomach problems of aspirin is to use enteric-coated aspirin (for example, Ecotrin). The enteric coating prevents disintegration of aspirin until it has passed through the stomach and entered the duodenum (the first part of the intestine), where a more favorable environment exists for dissolution of aspirin. Children and teenagers should not take aspirin for flulike illness, or for chicken pox, since this may trigger Reye's syndrome, a rare but serious illness associated with aspirin. Patients on blood thinners, such as Coumadin, should avoid aspirin (since aspirin itself prolongs bleeding time).

Those who cannot take aspirin can choose acetaminophen (Tylenol, Panadol) to lower fever and relieve pain. It can be used safely in children for flulike illnesses or with chicken pox. As with any medication, acetaminophen can have side effects. Tylenol is metabolized in the liver and should be carefully used by those with underlying liver abnormalities.

Sir William Osler, a world-renowned physician, once noted that "the desire to take medicine is perhaps the greatest feature which distinguishes man from animals." The truth of this statement is suggested by the scores of medications that are marketed for colds. Most of these products contain multiple ingredients, one or more of which have no legitimate role in relieving cold and sinus symptoms. A plain decongestant (Sudafed) will provide symptomatic relief for an uncomplicated cold. A decongestant-expectorant combination will also thin mucus in the nose and bronchial passages.

Decongestant-Expectorant Combinations

- Guaifed Syrup
- Robitussin Severe Congestion Liquid-Gels
- Robitussin PE Syrup
- Sudafed Non-Drying Sinus Liquid Caps
- Vicks Dayquil Sinus Pressure & Congestion Relief

COUGH PREPARATIONS

Cough is a symptom that frequently accompanies respiratory infections. Not all coughs are bad, since the cough itself is a protective reflex that helps clear secretions from the windpipe and bronchial tubes. Medications that suppress a cough relieve this annoying symptom and permit rest, but they have no direct effect on the underlying infection. Drinking warm liquids (tea, soup) and sucking on plain, hard candies are also helpful.

Nonprescription preparations that decrease the cough which may accompany respiratory infections are outlined in the Table 8.3. Some contain an antitussive (another word for anti-cough) alone; others also combine a decongestant.

Several other cough preparations that contain analgesics, antihistamines, and additional ingredients were not included. For most people with a cough that accompanies the common cold, one of the listed products should offer

TABLE 8.3   Over-the-counter Cough Preparations

PRODUCT	COUGH MEDICATION	DECONGESTANT
Cheracol D	X	
Cough-X Lozenges	X	
Delsym Cough Formula	X	
Dorcol Children's Cough Syrup	X	X
Halls Cough Drops	X	
Novahistine DMX	X	X
Pediacare Infant's Drops Decongestant Plus Cough	X	X
Pediatric Vicks 44D	X	X
Pediatric Vicks 44E	X	
Pertussin	X	
Robitussin Cough & Cold	X	X
Robitussin CF	X	X
Robitussin DM	X	
Ryna-C Liquid	X	
Ryna-CX Liquid	X	X
Sucrets	X	
Sudafed Children's Cold & Cough Liquid	X	X
Triaminic DM Cough & Decongestant Formula	X	X
Vicks 44D	X	X
Vicks 44E	X	

relief. In most cases, the cough preparation should loosen or thin mucus in the bronchial tubes. Cough medications containing antihistamines have not been listed, since antihistamines may have an undesirable drying effect. However, coughs associated with allergies such as hay fever or asthma will respond to antihistamines, but even in these cases the dryness produced may do more harm than good. There are a number of stronger antitussive products, which may contain codeine or other prescription drugs, for tougher-to-cure cases.

ANTIHISTAMINES: ANTI-ALLERGIC MEDICATIONS

Antihistamines are a group of drugs that have been used for more than fifty years to treat allergies. While these drugs are effective in a wide range of allergic problems, our discussion will focus on their use in treating nasal allergies. Since this book emphasizes self-help, those antihistamines that are available without a prescription will be stressed. In addition, you need some knowledge of prescription antihistamines in order to best utilize those that may be prescribed for your allergic symptoms.

An allergic reaction occurs when an offending substance, known as an allergen, comes in contact with the nasal lining of a person susceptible to that material, for example, when pollen grains are inhaled by someone with a ragweed allergy. This triggers the release of histamine, a chemical in our body that subsequently results in sneezing, congestion, and watery nasal drip characteristic of the allergic nasal reaction. Other allergic symptoms beyond the scope of this discussion may include watery eyes, itchy throat, cough, wheeze, and skin reactions. (Chapter 5 discusses allergy in detail.) Antihistamines compete with histamine at the cell surface and can prevent the histamine reaction that triggers allergic symptoms.

The antihistamines listed in Table 8.4 are available without a prescription.

TABLE 8.4   Antihistimines Available without a Prescription

GENERIC NAME	BRAND NAME	ANTIHISTAMINE PLUS DECONGESTANT
Diphenhydramine	Benadryl	Benadryl Allergy Decongestant Tablets
Clemastine Fumarate	Tavist	Tavist-D
Chlorpheniramine Maleate	Chlor-Trimeton	Chlor-Trimeton Allergy Decongestant Tablets
Brompheniramine	Dimetane	Dimetapp
Triprolidine		Actifed

Except for Tavist, which is available only in tablet form, the other antihistamines come in tablet or capsule form for adults and children twelve and older, and in liquid form for younger children. Consult the package for specific dosages. Some of the plain antihistamines and most of the antihistamine-decongestants are available in sustained-action dosages. This permits twice-a-day dosage rather than an every four–hour dose, as seen with some antihistamines. If your allergic symptoms primarily affect your eyes, a plain antihistamine should suffice. If these allergic symptoms are accompanied by a significant degree of nasal congestion or ear blockage, consider taking an antihistamine-decongestant combination. Remember that decongestants should be avoided in people with high blood pressure, heart disease, diabetes, thyroid disease, or by anyone taking a monoamine oxidase inhibitor.

There are several different classes of antihistamines. Benadryl and Tavist belong to one class of antihistamines; Chlor-Trimeton, Dimetane, and Actifed to another. If you do not get relief from one product, you should try one from the other group (rather than switching to one in the same group), since individuals may respond differently to each of the different groups. There are many combination antihistamines with different brand names from those listed, but almost all contain one of the generic antihistamines noted.

By far the most common side effect of antihistamines is their tendency to cause drowsiness. Other possible side effects include dry mouth, confusion, urinary retention, dizziness, and sedation. These side effects can be especially problematic in the elderly (including men with prostate problems), so antihistamines should be avoided by older patients if possible. When using an antihistamine-decongestant product, the drowsiness caused by the antihistamine may be counteracted by the excitement and stimulation caused by most decongestants. Children may paradoxically become excitable by antihistamines and may be unable to tolerate them.

Many other antihistamines are available only by prescription, and those will not be covered here. There are also a number of newer, non-sedating antihistamines, all of which can be obtained by prescription only. These have gained popularity in recent years, as evidenced by advertisements you may have seen. These include Allegra, Claritin and Claritin-D, Hismanal, and Seldane (Seldane has recently been taken off the market as a result of rare but serious cardiac side effects), and Zyrtec. Claritin has been touted to become a candidate for a future switch to nonprescription status. A new type of antihistamine, in the form of a nasal spray (called Astelin), has recently hit the market.

Antihistamines are best used to prevent allergy symptoms, which is medically termed as *prophylactic*. If you will be exposed to something that triggers your allergies, e.g., grass-cutting or animals, then take an antihistamine tablet one hour before exposure. After extended use, you may build up a tolerance to a given antihistamine. Switching to a different one, especially from a different class, may improve your response.

CORTICOSTEROIDS

ORAL STEROIDS

Corticosteroids (known as steroids), or cortisone, are wonder drugs with lifesaving ability in many medical disorders. They can also be overused by athletes and bodybuilders to increase muscle mass. With regard to the nose and sinuses, these drugs have potent anti-allergic and anti-inflammatory effects. They are frequently prescribed for one week to provide rapid reduction of an inflamed, swollen nasal lining and to improve sinus drainage. You can recognize cortisone, since it is usually prescribed in a tapering dosage, for example, six tablets the first day, five tablets the second day, four tablets the third day, etc. Cortisone tablets may be generic, such as Prednisone or Prednisolone, or a specific brand, such as Medrol or Decadron. Cortisone taken orally on an extended basis may result in serious side effects, such as gastrointestinal bleeding, weight gain with fluid retention, or personality change. If you have a history of stomach ulcers, high blood pressure, diabetes, or glaucoma, you should check with your doctor before taking any steroids, since they can exacerbate these conditions.

NASAL STEROID SPRAYS

Fortunately, many cortisone nasal sprays have been developed to provide relief of nasal congestion on a long-term basis. These nasal steroid sprays are not absorbed into the bloodstream, so they do not have the side effects listed for oral cortisone.

Nasal steroid sprays may take several or more days to take effect, so don't expect an immediate response. Decongestant nasal sprays (discussed earlier in this chapter) produce immediate nasal decongestion, but may result in rebound swelling of the nasal lining if used for more than a few days. Steroid sprays have the advantage of not causing rebound. If your nasal passages are extremely clogged, the prescribed spray may be ineffective because it cannot get past the nostrils. In this case, your physician may suggest oral medication to unclog the nose, after which the cortisone spray can be used effectively. For the best effect, direct the tip of the spray or aerosol device toward the side of your nose rather than toward its center.

Cortisone nasal sprays or aerosols are available only by prescription, but a knowledge of their mechanism of action and their side effects will be helpful if your doctor orders one for you. With the exception of the first cortisone aerosol available (Dexamethasone), those developed later act at the cell level within the nasal lining and are not absorbed into the body at a sufficient level to cause systemic (or bodily) side effects.

Side effects of cortisone sprays include nasal bleeding and nasal irritation or stinging. The latter symptoms tend to be transient and can often be prevented by first spraying the nose with saltwater (saline). This irritation is usually due to the vehicle rather than to the cortisone drug itself, so switching to a product with a different vehicle or delivery system may solve this problem. For example, some patients do better with the aqueous (water base) products. If bleeding develops, you may be advised to discontinue the spray for several weeks, then resume the steroid spray, using the saltwater before each dosage. With extended use (more than six months), some serious side effects, such as perforation (a hole) of the nasal septum, have been reported. Another theoretical side effect is fungal infection, which has been seen in the mouth after extended use with oral cortisone inhalers (used by asthmatics). Fortunately, fungal infection of the nose is rare. In any event, anyone using these sprays on a regular basis should be rechecked by the prescribing physician at least every four to six months. Prolonged, excessive use of steroid sprays could theoretically shut down the cortisone-producing center in the brain, but this has only been shown in animal studies

Currently Available Cortisone Nasal Sprays

- Beconase AQ Nasal Spray*

- Dexacort Aerosol

- Flonase

- Nasacort Nasal Inhaler; Nasacort AQ Spray

- Nasarel Nasal Solution

- Nasonex

- Rhinocort Nasal Inhaler

- Vancenase AQ Spray*; Vancenase Pockethaler

*AQ preparations are aqueous (mixed in water) and for some individuals, sting less in the nose.

with very high overuse of the drug. The steroid sprays may have potential harmful effects on a fetus, so if you are pregnant, avoid these or ask your obstetrician. Some of these nasal steroid sprays can be safely used for children six and older—although often at a lower dosage.

NASAL CROMOLYN SPRAY

Another prescription drug in a nasal spray (available orally and in a lung inhaler) is cromolyn sodium. This non-cortisone spray is effective in treating nasal allergies. You should be familiar with cromolyn nasal spray (brand name, Nasalcrom) since it has recently switched to over-the-counter status. The main action of this drug is to block the allergic reaction with release of histamine and other substances by sensitized cells in the nasal lining of an allergic person. Nasalcrom is most effective if used before exposure to an allergen, for example, just before the start of the pollen season. It has the advantage of not containing cortisone and can be used indefinitely, virtually without side effects. While cromolyn compares favorably with cortisone in its antiallergic effects, it is not as potent with regard to anti-inflammatory action. Another disadvantage of cromolyn spray is that it must be used at least four times a day as compared with the once- or twice-a-day dosage of most cortisone sprays. Cromolyn nasal spray (Nasalcrom) can be used with a high degree of safety in adults, and in children six and older. Despite the fact that some cortisone-containing nasal sprays have been approved for children six and older, parents are usually relieved if their children can be treated with a non-cortisone product.

ANTIBIOTICS

Antibiotics are prescription medications used to fight infections. They work by different mechanisms to destroy the bacteria that cause infections, and thus are usually prescribed by your doctor for sinus disease. There are different categories of antibiotics based on their chemical structures. Certain antibiotics work better for certain types of infections, but a complete discussion of this is beyond the scope of this book. However, I will outline the general categories of oral antibiotics that may be prescribed. New agents come out constantly, so at the time you read this, there may be additional drugs available.

The most common side effect of antibiotics are stomach upset and diarrhea, which can grow worse with long-term use. Eating yogurt (which contains active cultures)

Table 8.5 General Categories of Oral Antibiotics

GENERIC NAME	BRAND NAME
Penicillins	
amoxicillin	Amoxil
amoxicillin/clavulanate	Augmentin
ampicillin	Polycillin
dicloxacillin	Dynapen
penicillin	Pen-Vee K
*Cephalosporins**	
cefaclor	Ceclor
cefixime	Suprax
cefpodoxime	Vantin
cefprozil	Cefzil
cefuroxime axetil	Ceftin
cephalexin	Keflex
cephradine	Anspor, Velosef
loracarbef	Lorabid

Cephalosporins are derivatives of penicillins. Fewer than 10 percent of patients with a pencillin allergy will be allergic to cephalosporins.

Erythromycins and Other Macrolides	
azithromycin	Zithromax
clarithromycin	Biaxin
clindamycin	Cleocin

continued on next page

TABLE 8.5   *continued*

GENERIC NAME	BRAND NAME

Erythromycins and Other Macrolides
continued

erythromycin base, delayed release caps	Eryc
erythromycin base, film & enteric coated tablets	E-Mycin, Ery-Tub
erythromycin ethylsuccinate	EES, EryPED
erythromycin polymer coated partides	PCE
erythromycin stearate	Erythrocin
erythromycin with sulfa	Pediazole

Tetracyclines

doxycycline	Vibramycin, Monodox
minocycline	Minocin
tetracycline	Sumycin

Quinolones

ciprofloxacin	Cipro
ofloxacin	Floxin

Sulfas and Related/Combination Agents

sulfadiazine	Sulfadiazine
sulfamethoxazole/ trimethoprim	Bactrim DS, Septra DS

continued on next page

GENERIC NAME	BRAND NAME
Sulfas and Related/Combination Agents *continued*	
sulfisoxazole	Gantrisin
sulfisoxazole/erythromycin	Pediazole
Antifungal Agents*	
fluconazole	Diflucan

*These agents fight fungal infections (not bacterial infections), which are uncommonly involved in sinus disease.

daily or taking an acidophilus pill (found in health-food stores) can lessen these problems. Additionally, antibiotics fight bacteria but can therefore cause yeast infections (usually manifested as white thrush in the mouth, or vaginal itching). Again, yogurt and acidophilus can help prevent these. If stomach symptoms, diarrhea, or symptoms of a yeast infection persist, let your doctor know.

Many individuals are allergic to an antibiotic, manifested usually as a skin rash, or rarely as an anaphylactic reaction, with throat closing and breathing difficulty. An upset stomach as a reaction to a certain class of antibiotics can be helpful for your doctor to know but does not usually mean you are allergic to an antibiotic. Table 8.5 outlines the general classes of antibiotics. If you are allergic to one agent in the class, then you should avoid others in that category.

Long-term use of antibiotics has the potential harm of over-growth of resistant bacteria and more trouble fighting infections later, so they should be prescribed by your physician only when truly necessary.

Only oral antibiotics are listed, since these are primarily used for sinus infections. Intravenous antibiotics (administered by IV) are used in hospitalized patients with severe sinus infections or complications of sinus infections, such as orbital/eye abscess or brain infection. Rarely, a sinus infection can chronically infect the bone, necessitating a need for long-term IV antibiotics, which are given at home for several weeks. Of note, many of these oral antibiotics come in liquid form and can be used by children if prescribed by your doctor/pediatrician.

Oral antibiotics vary not only in their coverage of organisms but also in their price. Since these can be expensive, it is helpful to let your physician know whether you are paying out-of-pocket or are covered by a prescription plan with a co-pay.

CONCLUSION

This chapter has given an overview of the common classes of agents, with specific items listed, which are used to help sinus and nasal illness. Using the proper over-the-counter preparation should help relieve your symptoms and may help you avoid development of a full-blown sinus infection. Obviously, if you have a serious underlying medical condition, then you should contact your doctor first. In addition, persistent symptoms should prompt professional attention. The next chapter addresses what will occur upon seeking a physician's advice.

CHOOSING
A DOCTOR

This book has looked at sinus disease and other related problems. I hope you will be able to tell if you do, in fact, have a sinus problem and what may be causing it. Emphasis has been placed on nonprescription medications and other measures for providing easy relief. In some cases of nasal disease—for example, the common cold and mild allergies—self-treatment will be all that is necessary and may prevent full progression into a sinus infection. However, there will be times when you need the services of a physician. This chapter will review when you should seek professional medical care, what type of physician you should see, and what basic things these physicians will likely do for you.

WHEN TO SEE A DOCTOR

There are obvious times when you don't need to see a doctor and other times when you should definitely see one. For example, you don't need to run to the pediatrician every time your child has a sniffle—often, use of a humidifier or a few doses of an over-the-counter decongestant will suffice. And you probably don't need to see a doctor if once a year in the spring you have two days of sneezing, tearing eyes, and other allergy symptoms that are relieved with nonprescription antiallergy medications. On the other hand, when you have such a severe sinus infection that you have swelling and redness around one of your eyes or problems with your vision, it is fairly obvious that you need to see a doctor. But how about in-between cases? At what point should you see a physician?

It is difficult to outline every specific instance when a doctor's care should be sought, but I can give some general guidelines. If you have an underlying medical condition that makes it harder for you to fight infection, then you should see a doctor when your symptoms start, since there may be quicker progression of infection and possible complications of sinusitis. Examples of such individuals with sub-optimal immune systems against infection are people with diabetes, those on chemotherapy (anti-cancer) drugs, and patients who are HIV-positive or who have AIDS. A number of drugs purposely suppress the immune system, not allowing it to function properly. The most common of these is Prednisone, a form of steroid. When patients are on these medications, they are at risk for infections. Common situations in which steroids are used are in severe cases of asthma, rheumatoid arthritis, and after organ (kidney or heart) transplants.

Another group of people who should see a doctor sooner rather than later for nasal or sinus symptoms are patients with underlying lung diseases, such as asthma or emphysema. This is because lung problems can be worsened by a sinus infection; the infected mucus from the nose and sinuses can drip into the windpipe, bringing on an airway attack. For example, I see many asthmatics who only require lung inhalers (oral sprays for asthma) when they have a sinus infection. Once I am able to improve their sinus disease, their asthma attacks greatly improve, and they can cut back on their asthma meds.

There are also times when the otherwise healthy individual should see a doctor for their sinus symptoms. If your cold symptoms persist for more than seven to ten days, then you probably have a sinus infection, which may require an antibiotic (which only a doctor can prescribe) to clear up. Upper respiratory symptoms of the common cold were fully examined in Chapter 2, but when these progress to facial pain, fever, severe cough, or ear or throat discomfort, then it is time to visit a doctor for closer examination. While over-the-counter medications can be a great relief for your cold, allergy, and sinus symptoms, there are times when a stronger prescription medication is required to make you comfortable.

WHAT TYPE OF DOCTOR TO SEE

Once you have decided to seek a physician, what type of doctor should you see? For an otherwise healthy adult, the routine sinus infection can be treated by the family doctor or internist. Children should initially be evaluated by either a pediatrician or a family physician. Although the modern medical system has flourished as the result of specialization, the key to receiving good medical care lies with your general, family practitioner. He can manage most of the health problems you will face in your lifetime. The general practitioner should be able to direct you to a specialist when required.

In today's rapidly changing medical world, managed health care is becoming a stronger factor. These Health Maintenance Organizations, also known as HMOs, are composed of networks of primary-care physicians. Patients must see their primary doctor before being referred to a specialist. If you prefer to see a specialist at your own discretion, then you should choose an insurance plan that gives you such an option.

SEEING A SPECIALIST

If your sinus infections are sporadic and seem to easily clear up with an antibiotic, then you probably can be treated by your general practitioner. But once you start to develop symptoms of chronic sinusitis with recurring acute infections, prolonged infections, headaches, and nasal obstruction, it is time to see a specialist. Any patient with a sinus complication always needs specialist care. There are several types of physicians who commonly see sinus problems, each with a slightly different emphasis of treatment and care.

THE OTOLARYNGOLOGIST
(EAR, NOSE, AND THROAT DOCTOR)

The otorhinolaryngologist—a.k.a. the otolaryngologist or more commonly the ear, nose, and throat doctor—specializes in adult and pediatric diseases of the upper respiratory tract (the ears, nose, and throat). They treat patients both medically and surgically for sinus disease. After evaluation of your condition, an otolaryngologist will likely prescribe medications. When necessary, the ENT is able to perform procedures to "drain the sinuses" and correct anatomic abnormalities inside the nose through surgery. Some ENTs have an interest in allergy and may be involved in allergy-testing and shots.

THE ALLERGIST

The allergist is highly trained in management of allergies, including diagnosis through testing, and treatment with medications and shots. While not all sinus infections are caused by allergies, allergies do play a significant role in some chronic sinus disease. If you have severe allergic symptoms of thin, watery nasal discharge, sneezing, or tearing eyes, and if these seem to trigger sinus attacks, then you should probably see an allergist.

THE PULMONARY (LUNG) DOCTOR

There are a group of patients in whom chronic sinus disease is closely related to their lung problems. For example, some individuals develop asthma from thick postnasal drip and associated cough. Since they may require lung inhalers or other pulmonary medications, these patients are best treated by lung specialists, who can manage their lung disease, as well as the sinus infections that exacerbate their lung disease.

CHECKING CREDENTIALS

The general practitioner (GP) is a physician who, in the past, entered a medical practice after four years of medical school and one year of internship. Currently, the GP has been replaced by the family practitioner, who is certified by the American Academy of Family Practice upon successful completion of a three-year residency program. General practitioners already in practice could have obtained certification in family practice by passing a rigorous test. The family practice physician is trained to take care of the entire family unit—from children to the elderly. This compares with the internist (or internal medicine physician), who cares for adults only, or to the pediatrician, who sees only children.

All family practice physicians have to be recertified every seven years by passing a comprehensive test and accumulating a number of hours of postgraduate education each year. This ensures that physicians will keep up with future developments, a situation that had not been mandatory in the past. Many specialty groups also require that their members be reexamined and recertified periodically. Almost all physicians in this country are committed to spend one hundred fifty hours in postgraduate study every three years. Despite increasing criticism of physicians and hospitals, the overall training of physicians today is more comprehensive than it has ever been.

Candidly, I must admit that there is still a number of uninterested, poorly qualified physicians in practice today. The key to selecting a physician is to find one who is interested and ethical. Note the emphasis on "interested." Your physician must be interested, available, and able to communicate with you. Proficiency is important after these criteria are met. An honest family doctor should be able to refer you to a reputable specialist when the need arises.

In evaluating a physician, the term *board certified* indicates completion of the required years of postgraduate training following medical school, plus successful completion of tests—either written, practical, or both. A board-qualified physician is one who has completed the required number of years of training but has not yet passed the test needed for certification.

A specialist has additional training in his field of expertise. For example, the pulmonary (lung) specialist has two to three additional years of experience following three years of internal medicine training. The ear, nose, and throat surgeon begins with a surgical internship, followed by four to five additional years of specialty training.

Since any physician can designate himself a specialist, the best way to check his credentials is to ask if he is board certified or board qualified. Obviously, there are physicians competent to treat disease in which they have not received one of these designations; on the other hand, a passing score on a certification test doesn't guarantee competence or superior ability. But it is some assurance that the certified specialist has adequate preparation to practice his craft. Don't be afraid to ask your doctor about his credentials. A physician with good credentials welcomes the opportunity to show them off. If the doctor is offended by your questions, then consider looking elsewhere.

As society becomes more complex, so do the letters appended to a physician's name. The term *doctor* in front of a name is becoming generic, used by a whole variety of professionals who fall into the broad category of health-care providers. It may also be used by Ph.D.s, who have put long, hard years toward their degrees but are not in a position to treat illness (except for psychologists in the field of mental health).

The basic degree given by most medical schools in this category is M.D.—Doctor of Medicine. Several schools give a D.O. degree—Doctor of Osteopathy. For many years there was a rivalry between these two groups, with each using separate hospital facilities. Years ago much osteopathic theory of practice was based on manipulation of bones. Recently, osteopathic physicians have begun to receive comparable training to M.D.s and now practice along the same lines with regard to medical and surgical methods. In many states the two groups practice side by side, using the same hospital facilities.

After the letters M.D. or D.O. following a physician's name, you may see the designation F.A.A.F.P., F.A.C.S., F.A.C.P., or a similar set of initials. They stand for Fellow American Academy of Family Physicians; Fellow American College of Surgeons; and Fellow American College of Pediatricians, respectively. They imply membership in a specialty group, indicating successful completion of appropriate training and clinical experience. The physician with one of these ranks is a board-certified specialist. However, many other physicians have identical backgrounds but choose not to join the organization that permits them to add the appropriate letters to their name.

Another set of letters is being found with increasing frequency after a physician's name: P.C. Can you guess which specialty this signifies? None. P.C. stands for Professional Corporation. For the past few decades, physicians have been permitted to incorporate. This has nothing to do with the quality of health care provided, but is intended to allow physicians to take advantage of pension plans, profit sharing, group insurance, and other tax advantages open to industry for many years. If John Jones, M.D., wishes to incorporate, he must so signify by changing his office sign and stationery to John Jones, M.D., P.C.

In some physicians' offices or clinics you may be examined by Sam Smith, P.A. This stands for Physician's Assistant, a category of health personnel that is becoming popular in this country. Since many tasks performed by physicians can be carried out satisfactorily by someone with less training, many centers are now training physician's assistants. These highly motivated men and women work with a physician who directs their activity and assumes ultimate responsibility for the patient. Nurse practitioners may similarly work with some independence but under a physician's guidance.

WHEN CONSULTATION IS NEEDED

If your family physician suggests a consultation regarding your sinuses, ask for his guidance as to whom you should see (with many current insurance plans, you often need a written referral from your primary-care doctor). If you have previously dealt with a specialist in the field for your current problem, then mention this to your family doctor. If he still suggests a different consultant than you have named, you should probably go along with his advice. Most physicians will not criticize a colleague but are more likely to express their opinion by directing you to a more qualified person. Remember, in today's world of managed-care medicine, you may be limited to seeing a doctor in your plan unless you are willing to pay an additional fee.

There will be occasions when you have to go directly to a specialist or to make your own choice in this regard. Nurses, especially those who work at a hospital, make an excellent, unbiased source of information. They tend to be much more candid and often more knowledgeable about doctors than fellow physicians will be.

Another source of information about physicians is satisfied patients. When several neighbors, friends, or coworkers have been pleased with the services of a certain doctor, you feel more assured than by just picking a name out of the yellow pages or from a newspaper advertisement.

Most doctors have come to realize that today's patient wants to be well informed and to have some say in his treatment. The days of accepting whatever a doctor says as gospel are gone. Certainly you should feel at ease when talking with your physician, and hopefully your doctor can communicate freely with you rather than talking down to you.

When you are advised to have surgery, ask the following questions:

- "Are there alternative methods of treating this problem?"
- "What is the success rate of this operation?"
- "What are the risks of the surgery?"
- "How long is the recovery period?"

If the surgeon is not willing to frankly discuss these questions with you, then he may not be the doctor for you. Remember that in most circumstances surgery on the sinuses or nose is an elective procedure. You should feel comfortable in the recommendation for surgery, and that it is being offered as a last resort. If you have any hesitation, you may want to obtain a second opinion. Some medical-insurance plans will pay for this consultation, hoping that the money saved from unneeded surgery will more than make up the cost of these extra visits. You should not feel pressured to decide about surgery before you leave the doctor's office. The surgeon who urges you to make an immediate decision or who is too busy to answer your questions may be too busy to give your operation the attention it deserves. In this situation, you may want to seek a second opinion. Some of these details regarding surgery on the sinuses will be discussed in greater detail in the next chapter.

THE DOCTOR'S VISIT

Once you have decided to see a doctor for your sinus problem, what will he do? A competent physician should obtain a detailed history, including symptoms, past sinus problems, allergy symptoms, and general medical history. Examination of the head and neck area, as well as the lungs, is important. Some physicians, especially those who specialize in nasal and sinus problems, may use either a flexible or rigid scope to look into the nose to give a more complete view of the nasal anatomy. In some circumstances it is helpful to take what is known as a "culture." A sample of nasal mucus is collected and sent to a lab, where it is analyzed in terms of the type of organism it grows and what antibiotics will work best to kill the organism. This information may help your doctor prescribe an effective antibiotic. Cultures are especially useful in cases of persistent infection, or in patients with underlying medical conditions in which it is important to quickly eradicate the infection.

Your doctor may order an X ray of the sinuses. Although most sinus infections can be diagnosed by history and/or physical examination, there are times when a plain sinus film gives your doctor a way to better diagnose and follow an acute sinus infection. However, in the past decade plain sinus X-ray films have lost their popularity. CAT scans have become the gold standard study for sinus disease. These involve sitting in a machine for roughly fifteen minutes, and the pictures obtained show multiple slices through the brain and sinuses. This scan gives an excellent view of all four sets of sinuses, with emphasis on the underlying bony structures. Although a CAT scan should not be ordered at the first sign of a sinus infection, it is useful in assessing cases of prolonged or recurrent infection. The CAT scan allows your doctor to examine for any underlying bony abnormalities that predispose to sinus disease (and which may possibly be corrected surgically). The CAT scan is a necessity in cases of a sinus complication, such as an orbital (eye) problem, since it provides exquisite detail of the eye and allows for assessment of a possible abscess, which would require immediate surgical drainage.

Another sophisticated X-ray study is the MRI scan. The MRI is better for soft-tissue and brain abnormalities, and is typically not useful for sinus disease. It is an overly sensitive study in which even a mild cold will show sinus-tissue swelling. As an ear, nose, and throat specialist, I am often referred patients who have had an MRI scan for another reason and may have sinus swelling on their scan. Unless they are having sinus symptoms, these findings are usually of no significance. On the other hand, there are times when an MRI is useful for sinus problems. If there is a concern of a possible sinus tumor, an MRI is helpful in outlining the tumor from surrounding infection. The MRI is also helpful in those cases where the sinus disease may involve the brain structures or the lining around the brain, called the meninges (for example, in cases of brain abscess or meningitis).

CONCLUSION

After your doctor has obtained a history, examined you, and possibly cultured or X-rayed your sinuses, it is time for treatment. This usually consists of medications, typically antibiotics to fight infection, and decongestants (oral and nasal sprays), and antihistamines (for allergy symptoms) when needed. Chapter 8 gave a detailed look at the classes of medications available for sinus disease. When allergy is a strong contributor to your sinus problems, allergy shots might be recommended. When all else fails, surgery is an option for chronic sinus disease, or for cases in which there is an anatomic abnormality underlying recurrent nasal problems. The next chapter will further explore surgical options for treating sinus disease.

SINUS SURGERY

O nce you have tried home remedies, taken over-the-counter, as well as prescription medications, and have had multiple visits to your doctor for sinus infections, it may be time to consider surgical options. Take, for example, my patient Pat, a baby-sitter who for two years had monthly sinus infections, which usually required two ten-day courses of an antibiotic to clear up. She awoke almost daily with a sinus headache that lasted most of the day and made work difficult. Her nose was always blocked, and her husband reported that her snoring had become so loud he slept in a different room. Despite two months of antibiotics, nasal steroid sprays, and decongestants, her symptoms persisted. When allergy testing was negative and her CAT scan showed infection and blockage in all her sinuses, Pat and I decided it was time for surgery.

This chapter will examine trends in current surgical treatment for sinusitis. It will help you determine if you, like Pat, might benefit from sinus surgery. This should help you to better understand when you may be a surgical candidate and what you can expect from your surgery.

INDICATIONS FOR SINUS SURGERY

Most surgical procedures for sinus disease are usually elective. What I usually tell my sinus patients is that they have three options with long-standing sinus disease: (1) do nothing; (2) take medications; or (3) have surgery. There are only a few particular situations, which we will later discuss, in which surgery on the sinuses is required to prevent major complications. Most of the time, sinus surgery is performed for a chronic sinus infection that is not responding to antibiotics, or for multiple recurrent acute infections. In general, most sinus infections are not life-threatening but can greatly alter the quality of life with persistent headaches, nasal blockage, and cough. Thus, the decision to have surgery for your sinus problems is ultimately up to you, the patient.

Although surgery today is safe, with a fairly easy recovery, there are always risks involved with any procedure. It is wise to feel that you have exhausted all other options prior to surgery. This should include at least four to six weeks of antibiotics, prescription nasal sprays, decongestants, and possibly antihistamines and steroids. Only you can determine the severity of your symptoms and the improvements with medical therapy. Obviously, your philosophy toward surgery may be different if you are twenty-one and healthy, versus if you are sixty-one with many other medical problems. Your surgeon may guide you in terms of when he feels that surgery is indicated, but you should feel that you have made an informed decision yourself.

There are times when a surgical option is definitely indicated. A tumor, especially if malignant, requires at least a biopsy and possibly complete surgical removal (while some tumors respond to surgery, others respond to radiation and chemotherapy medications). Patients with underlying medical problems that are worsened by their sinusitis often benefit greatly from sinus surgery. One example of this is the asthma patient, whose lung symptoms flare up because of sinus infection and postnasal drip. My patient Bill was an asthmatic on three different inhalers, as well as oral medications including steroids. Once I drained his sinuses and removed chronically infected tissue, he was able to stop all medications and use only one inhaler on an as-needed basis.

There may also be the severely ill intensive care–unit patient, who is at increased risk for sinus infection and may require sinus drainage for full treatment. Because the sinuses sit near the eye and brain, there are rare complications involving these areas, requiring immediate drainage to prevent visual loss, brain infection, or brain abscess. Patients with poor immune systems, such as the cancer patient on chemotherapy, may become ill with a sinus infection and may require drainage (sometimes only for a culture to determine the exact organism causing the infection and aid in choosing the appropriate antibiotic).

Whether nasal polyps need to be removed is still debatable—even among ear, nose, and throat surgeons.

159

Since most polyps are noncancerous, some doctors feel that if not symptomatic, they can be watched. Other physicians believe that polyps should at least be biopsied to rule out that they are not cancerous or precancerous. In general, if you have polyps that persist even after medication (cortisone by mouth and/or by nasal spray), surgical removal is usually worthwhile to improve nasal symptoms.

Once you and your doctor have decided that you are a surgical candidate, what are your options? A variety of sinus procedures is used for different situations. We will review the more common procedures carried out for sinus disease today to give you an idea of when each procedure is best utilized, and what exactly each procedure involves.

SURGERY FOR ACUTE SINUSITIS

Most cases of an acute sinus infection involving nasal discharge, congestion, and facial pressure respond to oral medications. This typically includes an antibiotic for ten to fourteen days, an oral or topical decongestant, or an oral steroid. Sometimes the facial pain and pressure is so severe that the patient may require a prescription pain medication. For the patient with persistent, unrelenting symptoms of an acute sinus infection, a sinus irrigation to flush or drain the affected sinus(es) can provide relief. This was more commonly performed in the past, with younger physicians not frequently employing this technique.

Sinus irrigation is carried out in the ENT physician's office, using local anesthesia (i.e., novocaine). An instrument is placed in the maxillary sinus and the sinus flushed with sterile saltwater. Another, older technique is that of

Proetz displacement, in which a pressurized saltwater irrigation is combined with suctioning to displace infected material from the sinuses. These techniques to drain the sinuses can be uncomfortable but can help clear a painful, acute sinus infection. In addition, they allow the doctor to obtain material from inside the sinus to see what is growing. This helps the doctor choose the most appropriate antibiotic. However, in recent years nasal telescopes, called endoscopes, have gained great popularity. They allow for thorough examination inside the nose, where a specimen of pus can be obtained from a sinus opening (ostium), grown for culture, and a specific antibiotic chosen.

Two types of acute sinus infection merit special attention: An acute infection of the frontal (forehead) or sphenoid (behind the eyes) sinus—each of which sits particularly near to the brain—are considered more serious and require close care. If several days of oral antibiotics don't work, then the patient should receive intravenous medications in the hospital. When several days of IV antibiotics fail to improve the situation, surgical drainage of the sinus should be considered.

For the sphenoid sinus, drainage can be carried out through the nose, where the sinus is opened and pus is drained. Acute frontal sinus infections can be drained through the nose, where the sinus empties. Another way to drain the frontal sinus is externally through an incision under the eyebrow. This is called a frontal sinus trephination, and is performed in the operating room. After the eyebrow incision is made, a hole is made through the bone into the frontal sinus to allow for wide drainage. This leaves a small scar that typically heals well.

SURGERY FOR CHRONIC SINUSITIS

The most common reason that the sinuses are operated on is chronic infection. When symptoms become so severe and are not improving with medications, it is time to consider surgery.

In the past, the sinuses were approached externally through incisions on the face to clear chronic infection. The idea was to remove the chronically infected material from within the sinus and strip the tissue lining the sinus to clear infection. Although these techniques are still sometimes used, in recent years surgery is usually carried out through the nose. However, we will review these previous techniques, since you may have undergone them prior to the early 1990s. Additionally, external procedures are useful for removing large polyps, tumors, or for patients who have already undergone intranasal (through the nose) surgery.

A frequently infected sinus is the maxillary sinus. In the past, this sinus was usually approached through an incision under the upper lip through the gum, a procedure called a Caldwell-Luc operation. After a cut is made in the gum, the cheek sinus is entered by making a hole in its front wall and directly stripping out the disease. Patients can usually leave the hospital the day of surgery, with mild pain and swelling. The Caldwell-Luc is still employed, especially in cases with large maxillary sinus disease, which is difficult to remove through the nose.

The ethmoid sinuses (between the eyes) can be drained externally through an incision in the skin. This is often employed when the sinus infection is so severe that it leads to infection around the eye or to an eye abscess. Although there is an external scar on the face, the eye is seen directly during the surgery and is thus kept safe from injury. If you had sinus surgery years ago and have a small scar near your eye, chances are that you underwent an external ethmoidectomy, meaning removal of the ethmoid sinuses through an incision made on the outside of the face as opposed to going internally or intranasally through the nose.

Several operations are employed to get rid of chronic disease of the frontal or forehead sinus. Since this sinus drains into the nose through a small opening called the nasofrontal duct (going from the frontal sinus into the nose), it is prone to blockage and chronic infection despite intranasal surgery. The frontal sinus can be drained externally through an incision under the eyebrow. This allows the surgeon to look into the sinus and widen the opening of the frontal sinus into the nose.

Sometimes, however, disease of the frontal sinus persists despite this type of drainage. As a last resort for unresponsive disease, your surgeon may recommend a frontal sinus obliteration, in which the lining membrane of the frontal sinus is stripped and the sinus cavity packed with fat from the belly to close off the sinus. In rare cases of brain infection or abscess from frontal sinus infection, this or a similar procedure is utilized. The incision for this type of surgery is made in the hair, with the scalp pulled forward to expose the forehead, causing little cosmetic deformity. However, it is a relatively extensive procedure and should be recommended only in cases of prolonged disease that has failed all other modalities of treatment.

ENDOSCOPIC SINUS SURGERY

Since the mid 1980s, the surgical appproach to sinus disease in the United States has seen great change. Today, roughly two hundred thousand sinus surgeries are performed yearly in the United States, and most of these are carried out through the nose by a procedure called functional endoscopic sinus surgery. (This is also known as endoscopic sinus surgery, FESS, or just ESS.) Telescopes are used in the nose for visualization, leading to a simpler recovery for the patient. FESS not only refers to the specific procedure but also to a newer philosophy in dealing with chronic sinusitis.

Roughly twenty to thirty years ago, the focus was on the individual sinuses that became infected. This was predominantly the frontal and the maxillary sinuses, which showed up well on plain films and had significant symptoms of forehead and cheek pain. Surgeries focused on treating these sinuses, and thus the popularity of the Caldwell-Luc, external frontal drainage, and frontal sinus obliteraton. It was believed that if the sinuses were blocked, then they needed to drain dependently (from high to low). This popularized the so-called "nasal-antral window," an opening at the floor of the maxillary sinus (also known as the antrum) into the nose.

In the past two decades a much better understanding of sinus physiology has developed (see Chapter 1 for a more complete explanation). The sinuses drain via the ostiomeatal complex (the OMC).

Even minor changes in the OMC, which lies in the ethmoid chamber, can lead to subsequent blockage of the maxillary, frontal, and sphenoid sinuses. Assuming a patient has normal mucociliary clearance and can move mucus through the nose with properly functioning hair cells, then if the OMC is clear, the sinuses should drain correctly. With the increased use of CAT scans and nasal endoscopes, disease of this ostiomeatal complex can be identified. Attention during surgery is directed at his OMC rather than at the secondarily infected frontal and maxillary sinuses.

The aim of endoscopic sinus surgery is to relieve obstruction in the nose and at the ostiomeatal complex to allow for normal sinus drainage. This is done with minimal removal of tissue. Using endoscopes through the nose, thickened and diseased tissue that blocks the sinus ostia is removed. Most of the tissue from within the sinus, however, is maintained. This allows for a more rapid restoration of normal mucociliary flow and healthy sinuses after surgery.

ADJUNCTIVE PROCEDURES

Several other conditions may contribute to sinus disease and can be addressed at the same time as endoscopic surgery is carried out on the nose. Polyps (which are inflammatory growths covered more fully in Chapter 4), often block the sinus openings and lead to infection. Removal can be carried out with the use of endoscopes in conjunction with endoscopic sinus surgery. The midline structure called the septum in the nose can be twisted (known as a deviated septum) to the point that it restricts flow from the sinuses, with secondary infection. In these cases, when the sinuses are being treated surgically, the septum should also be straightened (see Chapter 4 for details) to alleviate the underlying culprit.

Surgery inside the nose should have no effect on the patient's appearance. However, external, cosmetic surgery on the nose can be performed in conjunction with internal work. This typically requires an additional, out-of-pocket fee, since plastic surgery is not covered by your insurance company.

WHAT TO EXPECT FROM
ENDOSCOPIC SINUS SURGERY

The use of endoscopes to perform sinus surgery has simplified things for the patient. The procedure, typically performed at a hospital or surgery center, takes roughly one to three hours depending upon the extent of work to be done. It can be done under either general anesthesia or local anesthesia with IV sedation with medication to make you drowsy, as well as novocainelike medication in your nose. While local anesthesia is less risky and offers fewer complications and an easier recovery, some surgeons prefer that their patients be "all the way asleep" with general anesthesia. What type of anesthesia is best for you should be discussed with your doctor prior to surgery, since every case is different and depends on your surgeon, the extent of your sinus disease, and your underlying medical problems. One tip I find that helps my patients tolerate sedation more easily, especially since I am working near the face, is to have them listen to a tape via a portable tape player.

Most patients are able to go home on the same day as their endoscopic sinus surgery. However, if you have any underlying medical problems, such as heart disease, asthma, or diabetes, your doctor may prefer you stay in the hospital overnight following your procedure. Usually some gauze or other type of packing is placed in the nose after surgery, and is left in place for one to five days. There is no external cast placed, unless cosmetic work has been done in conjunction with your sinus surgery. Similarly, there is no swelling or bruised eyes except for cosmetic cases, in which the nose must often be rebroken.

After endoscopic sinus surgery, it may take several weeks to months to fully heal. There is dry blood, mucus, and crusting in the nose, presenting symptoms of a severe cold or sinus infection. Most physicians recommend salt-water sprays or irrigations to decrease scabbing, along with antibiotic lubricant ointments (for example, Bacitracin or Polysporin ointment). Some surgeons keep their patients on oral antibiotics and oral steroids as they are healing. A prescription painkiller (such as Tylenol with codeine) may be required in some individuals to lessen discomfort. While most people can return to work several days after endoscopic sinus surgery, heavy activity and exercise should be avoided for at least two weeks in order to prevent scabs from falling off, and subsequent bleeding. Medications such as aspirin or ibuprofen (for example, Advil or Motrin) cannot be used for several weeks post-op, since these lead to thinning of the blood and increase the chance of bleeding. Tylenol-containing products, on the other hand, are safe in this regard. Remember, these are only rough guidelines to follow in terms of postoperative care after intranasal sinus surgery; every surgeon has his own set of rules.

Most surgeons feel that an integral part of endoscopic sinus surgery is the postoperative care. This not only includes local irrigations by the patient but also cleaning out of the nose and sinus cavities by the doctor in his office.

This helps to prevent scar formation, as well as facilitates healthy sinus healing. This process of cleaning out the sinus cavities is called debridement, in which the doctor, in his office, begins by numbing the inside of your nose with sprays or injections. He then uses the endoscope for visualization to clean out the nose and sinuses, removing crusts, scabs, and dry mucus. This is believed to be a key factor for a successful result from surgery. While every surgeon's post-op routine varies, most see their patients every one to three weeks after surgery until healing is complete, in four to ten weeks.

RISKS OF
ENDOSCOPIC SINUS SURGERY

While endoscopic sinus surgery has proved successful in most cases of chronic sinus problems, like any other surgical procedure, it is not without risks. Although these risks are rare, you should weigh the benefits of the surgery. With any surgical procedure, there is always a risk of the anesthesia medications. If you have any significant underlying medical problem, check with your general doctor to make sure you are in good enough general health to undergo a surgical procedure. Bleeding and infection may occur after sinus surgery but typically not to any severe extent.

Scar tissue can form in the nose and may require further treatment. Your surgeon would need to cut and remove any scar bands if they are affecting sinus drainage.

There are two particular complications of sinus surgery, which are rare but can be debilitating if they occur: Since the sinuses sit near the brain and the eyes, these structures are at risk of injury during surgery. These problems occur infrequently, but nonetheless will be described by your doctor as a "possible risk."

One group of patients who should be particularly cautious prior to undergoing sinus surgery are professional singers or others whose livelihood depends on their voice. There has been no definite answer yet as to whether there is a change in vocal resonance from alterations made in the sinus cavities as a result of surgery. Thus, any nasal procedure in these individuals should be undertaken as a last resort.

Probably the most commonly occurring problem after endoscopic sinus surgery is recurrent or persistent disease. In some patients, there may be scarring or other anatomic reasons for failure, which can be corrected. In others, however, there may be underlying nasal mucosal problems contributing to sinus infections. Despite a well-healed surgical sinus cavity, persistent disease of the nasal and sinus tissues may remain. This can be seen in highly allergic individuals, or in asthmatics who have diseased respiratory tissue. If you fall into one of these categories, you should not expect miracles from your surgeon. Instead, you should hope for control of your nasal problems, with topical sprays or perhaps a short course of antibiotics when needed for an acute infection. For some people, the goal of sinus surgery is not for cure but for better control of their problems.

WHAT ABOUT LASERS?

In the 1990s, lasers have become a marketing tool for medical procedures. While in some cases of bony growths, scarring, or polyps they may prove useful, they are by no means a standard or even a benefit for the typical sinus surgical case. For sinus surgery, lasers are more a gimmick for attracting patients, without much (if any) advantage over standard techniques.

CONCLUSION

This chapter should help you understand some of the basic surgical procedures now employed for sinus disease. While most patients with sinusitis can be treated with medications, there are times when surgery is indicated. You should be able to tell—with the help of your doctor— whether you would benefit from sinus surgery. The key to a successful surgery includes reasonable expectations, which this chapter has attempted to provide.

RESOURCES

NASAL AND SINUS IRRIGATION KITS

As described in Chapter 3, saline (saltwater) sprays can be helpful in preventing and relieving upper respiratory and sinus infections. In addition to the various over-the-counter sprays mentioned in the book, a number of commercial kits and irrigation systems can provide further relief. Steam-inhalation systems can be useful for chronic sinus sufferers. Many of these products are also useful after sinus surgery to help with healing, cleaning the nose and sinus passages of crusts and dry blood postoperatively. Below is a list of some of these products, including addresses and phone numbers of the companies that offer them.

Grossan Sinus Irrigation
Hydro Med, Inc.
phone: 1-800-560-9007
e-mail: hydromed@westworld.com
website: http://www.ent-consult.com

This is a special irrigator tip hooked up to a water pic system for sinus irrigation.

LAVAGE (Sinusitis Treatment Kit)
LAVAGE
8602 E. Whitewater Dr., Suite #210
Anaheim Hills, CA 92808
phone: 1-800-6-LAVAGE
fax: 714-627-9228

This kit includes a syringe and bottle system for sinus cleaning. A measuring spoon and cup are included for making normal saline (saltwater).

Magellan Steam Inhaler
The Magellan Group's Tools for Living
Dept. TMY971
2515 East 43rd Street
P.O. Box 182236
Chattanooga, TN 37422
phone: 1-800-644-8100 ext. TMY971
website: http://www.tmgusa.com

A steam inhaler that can be used by children and adults.

PRETZ (Irrigation)
Parnell Pharmaceuticals, Inc.
P.O. Box 5130
Larkspur, CA 94977
phone: 1-800-45-PHARM
fax: 415-256-8099
email: mail@parnellpharm.com

Pretz is a saline solution with glycerin and natural Yerba Santa for additional lubrication of nasal and sinus cavities. The irrigation product allows for irrigation of the Pretz solution.

> *RhinoFlow (Micronized E.N.T. Wash)*
> Respironics (Always Thinking)
> 1001 Murray Ridge Drive
> Murrysville, PA 15668-8550
> phone: 1-800-345-6443 or 412-733-0200
> fax: 412-733-0299
> website: http://www.respironics.com

A system that aerosolizes solutions for nasal irrigation and humidification. Allows for aerosol steam to be delivered to the nasal cavity and sinuses.

ASTHMA AND ALLERGY GROUPS

As explained in Chapters 3 and 5, allergy and asthma are closely linked to sinus disease. Below is a list of several self-help groups and educational resources for further information on these conditions.

> *Allergy and Asthma Network/Mothers of Asthmatics*
> 3554 Chain Bridge Road
> Suite 200
> Fairfax, VA 22030-2709
> phone: 703-385-4403

> *AllerDays Resource Center*
> phone: 1-800-595-3139
> website: http://www.allerdays.com

A program sponsored by Hoechst Marion Roussel pharmaceutical company, with educational materials for management of allergies.

Asthma Control Program
phone: 1-800-732-3364

Glaxo Wellcome pharmaceutical company sponsors this kit. It includes an Asthma Control booklet, a special medical ID card, a daily tracker to record symptoms, and other useful tools.

Clear Relief Allergy Line
phone: 1-800-522-7300

Schering Laboratories provides a free video ("Children and Allergy"), plus allergy-relief information.

GLOSSARY

Adenoids
Tissue that sits in the nasopharynx. Present in children, it shrinks by the late teens and early twenties.

Allergens
Substances that trigger an allergic response.

Allergic Rhinitis
Inflammation of the nose secondary to allergy.

Allergy
Hypersensitivity to a specific substance that does not cause symptoms in most people.

Analgesic
Medication that helps to relieve pain.

Anaphylaxis
Allergic reactions that occur immediately and progress rapidly; can be life-threatening.

Antibiotic
Medication that fights against bacterial infection.

Antihistamine
Medication that fights allergy symptoms.

Antitussive
Medication designed to relieve coughing.

Asthma
Disease in which there is a lower lung airway sensitivity to a variety of stimuli.

CAT Scan
A type of X ray—Computerized Axial Tomography—which shows multiple slices through the area of interest.

Choanal Atresia
Condition, congenital in origin, in which there is complete blockage at the back of one or both nostrils.

Choanal Stenosis
Condition in which there is narrowing in the back of one or both nostrils.

Cilia
Microscopic hairs that line the respiratory passages and help to propel the overlying mucus blanket.

Cluster Headache
Intense, one-sided headaches which can be accompanied by tearing and watery nasal discharge; associated with dilated blood vessels.

Cold
Viral infection of the nose and surrounding upper respiratory passages.

Common Cold
See cold.

Concha Bullosa
Enlargement of a middle turbinate by an air cell trapped within; this may block normal sinus drainage and can cause headache.

Corticosteroids
See steroids.

Cortisone
See steroids.

CT Scan
See CAT scan.

Cystic Fibrosis
Hereditary disease consisting of abnormal gland function. It is found mostly in children, who get digestive, lung, sinus, and nasal polyp disease.

Decongestant
An oral medication or nasal spray which opens the nasal passages by shrinking the lining of the nose.

Desensitization
A program of allergy injections designed to raise a patient's immunity to allergens.

Deviated Septum
A twist of the central nasal septum, that may narrow the nasal airway and require surgical correction.

Eczema
A skin condition with redness, swelling, crusting, scaling, and itching.

Endoscopic Sinus Surgery
A surgical procedure in which the sinuses are operated on via the nose using an endoscope (telescope) for visualization.

Eosinophils
A type of blood cell that is increased during an allergic response.

Eustachian Tube
A tube that runs between the nasopharynx and the ear, equalizing pressure between them.

Functional Endoscopic Sinus Surgery
See Endoscopic Sinus Surgery.

Gastroesophageal Reflux
A condition in which stomach acids back up into the esophagus (food pipe); often associated with a hiatal hernia.

Halitosis
Medical term for bad breath.

Histamine
Substance in the body which triggers a full-blown allergic reaction.

Immunoglobulin
A class of proteins that the body produces to help fight infections.

Immuno-suppressed
Condition of a poorly functioning immune system which fights infection; can occur in patients with HIV, AIDS, transplant patients, and cancer patients undergoing chemotherapy.

Interferon
A protein material, still somewhat experimental, that can act to ward off viral attacks.

Migraine
A type of headache caused by distension of the blood vessels in the head which is severe and recurrent.

MRI

A type of X ray—Magnetic Resonance Imaging—which takes multiple slices through the area of interest without using radiation.

Mucolytic

A type of medication which thins mucus so it can be more easily cleared from the respiratory tract.

Myalgia

Pain caused by muscular discomfort.

Nasal Cycle

The normal process whereby each side of the nose alternately opens and closes.

Nasal Smear

A sample of nasal secretions collected and analyzed in a laboratory.

Nasopharynx

Area located in the back of the nose.

Neuralgia

Pain that occurs when a nerve fires abnormally and produces pain in the area supplied by the nerve.

Olfaction

Sense of smell.

Ostiomeatal Complex (OMC)

Central area located in the ethmoid sinuses through which all the sinuses drain; when this area is blocked, other sinuses become secondarily infected.

Ostium

The opening of a sinus where it drains into the nose.

Otolaryngologist
Physician specializing in diagnosis and treatment of ear, nose, throat, and head and neck disorders. Also called an otorhinolaryngologist.

Paranasal Sinus
Air-filled bony cavities located adjacent to the nose in the face and skull.

Perennial Allergies
Allergies which occur throughout the year.

Polyp
Grapelike, inflammatory swelling of the nasal and sinus linings.

Pulmonologist
Physician specializing in diagnosis and treatment of lung diseases.

RAST (radioallergosorbent test)
An allergy blood test which measures specific antibodies which are produced in response to certain allergens.

Rhinitis
Inflammation of the lining of the nose.

Seasonal Allergies
Allergies which produce symptoms during particular seasons of the year.

Septum
Bony and cartilaginous partition that separates the right and left sides of the nose.

Sinuses
See paranasal sinus.

Sinusitis
Inflammation of the lining of one or more of the paranasal sinuses.

Steroids

A type of medication that can be used for nasal and sinus problems for its strong anti-allergy and anti-inflammatory effects; same as cortisone or corticosteroids.

Temporomandibular Joint (TMJ)

Joint where the jaw hinges in front of each ear; can be a source of headache.

Tension Headache

Most common type of chronic headache. The headache has a tight, "bandlike" quality to it; often associated with anxiety and depression.

Tic Douloureux

See Trigeminal Neuralgia.

Trigeminal Neuralgia

A pain that is severe, sharp, spasmodic, and occurs in any part of the face. Also known as tic douloureux.

Turbinates

Bones located on the side wall of the nose; there are three turbinates on each side of the nose—the inferior, middle, and superior.

Upper Respiratory Infection (URI)

An infection involving the lining of the nose or throat, usually viral in origin.

Vaccine

A preparation which is injected into the body and allows the body's immune system to make antibodies that will fight against a specific ailment.

BIBLIOGRAPHY

"Allergic Rhinitis and Sinusitis: Causation and Outcomes." *Clinical Courier, American Academy of Otolaryngic Allergy Foundation* 5, no. 4 (March 1997).

Anderson-Parrado, Patricia. "Relieve Colds and Allergies with Homeopathic Remedies." *Better Nutrition* 59, no. 3: 26 (March 1997).

Current Therapy in Otolaryngology, Head and Neck Surgery, 5th ed. (St. Louis: Mosby-Year Book, Inc., 1994).

"Diagnosis and Management of Acute and Chronic Sinusitis." *University of Virginia Reports on Respiratory Infections* 1, no. 1 (1997).

Farb, Stanley N. *The Ear, Nose, and Throat Book.* (New York: Appleton-Century-Crofts, 1980).

"Inflammatory Diseases of the Sinus." *Otolaryngic Clinics of North America* 26, no. 4 (August 1993).

Krause, Helen F., M.D. *Otolaryngic Allergy and Immunology.* (Philadelphia: W.B. Saunders Company, 1989).

"Medical Management of Sinusitis: Educational Goals and Management Guidelines." *Annals of Otology, Rhinology & Laryngology* 104, no. 10: part 2 (October 1995).

"Otolaryngic Allergy." *Otolaryngic Clinics of North America* 25, no. 1 (February 1992).

"Pediatric Sinusitis." *Otolaryngic Clinics of North America* 29, no. 1 (February 1996).

"Primer on Allergic and Immunologic Diseases." *Journal of the American Medical Association* 268, no. 20 (November 25, 1992).

Settipone, Guy A. *Rhinitis,* 2d ed. (Providence, R.I.: Ocean Side Publications, Inc., 1991).

Springen, Karen. "Get the Cold Facts." *Country Journal* 23, no. 5: 12 (Sept–Oct 1996).

INDEX